CLINICAL EFFECTIVENESS MADE EASY

First thoughts on clinical governance

Ruth Chambers

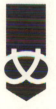

Staffordshire
UNIVERSITY

RADCLIFFE MEDICAL PRESS

©1998 Ruth Chambers
Illustrations ©1998 Martin Davies

Radcliffe Medical Press Ltd
18 Marcham Road, Abingdon, Oxon OX14 1AA

British Library Cataloguing in Publication Data

A catalogue record for this book is available from the British Library.

ISBN 1 85775 316 X

Typeset by Advance Typesetting Ltd
Printed and bound by TJ International Ltd, Padstow, Cornwall

► CONTENTS

► ABOUT THE AUTHOR

Ruth Chambers has been a general practitioner for 17 years. She is currently Professor of Health Commissioning at the School of Health, Staffordshire University. Her interest in clinical effectiveness and clinical audit grew during her three-year spell as Chairman of Staffordshire Medical Audit Advisory Group until 1996.

Ruth has run several series of clinical effectiveness workshops, teaching a mix of primary and community care health professionals clinical effectiveness skills in easy steps. The experiences of those workshops have informed this book.

► ACKNOWLEDGEMENTS

The workshops and composition of this book were developed with a grant from the regional Evidence-supported Medicine Union (EMU) to improve evidence-based care in the West Midlands.

North Staffordshire Medical Audit Advisory Group were joint organizers of the workshop series.

The book is based upon the experiences from running two series of four workshops, *Clinical Effectiveness Made Easy*, for primary and community care practitioners. I am grateful to the participants of the workshops for contributing so many ideas and being such an enthusiastic bunch of health professionals. Irene Fenton, the medical librarian, provided the inspiration and clear advice about undertaking literature searches and other sources of evidence.

I am grateful to my husband Chris for doing all the searches, Nicky Macleod for her contribution about the meaning of cost-effectiveness, and my colleagues who helped to facilitate the workshops.

Ruth Chambers
August 1998

This book is dedicated to those who think that clinical effectiveness is a 'good thing' but have no evidence for that assumption.

Clinical effectiveness is about knowing what you should be doing and being able to put that knowledge into practice

Overall aim of the programme

To increase awareness of, and skills in, the adoption of an evidence-based approach to the practice and delivery of health care.

Objectives of this book

This programme is for all health professionals to learn how to:

► ask the right question – it must be important to you and your colleagues
► look for the evidence and do a library search
► receive and incorporate constructive criticism from colleagues about their developing questions and search for evidence
► select the best evidence – what to do where none exists
► evaluate and interpret the evidence, such as read and extract information from a report
► apply the evidence as appropriate in a practice, unit or department

▶ act on the evidence to improve the practice of clinical effectiveness
▶ plan for clinical governance.

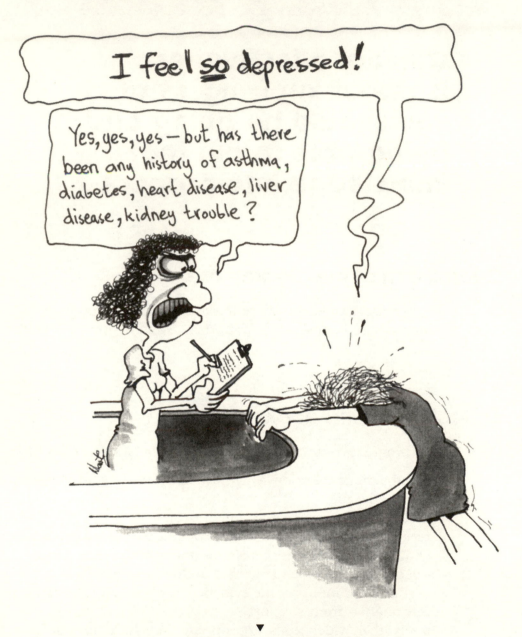

Do you need to update your style of practice?

Self-assessment of where you are now with clinical effectiveness

Before you start working through the clinical effectiveness programme, assess your baseline knowledge and attitudes to the topic. Please circle as many answers as apply, or fill in the information requested.

1 How confident do you feel that you are capable of practising clinical effectiveness to be able to:

ask a relevant question?	*Very*	*Somewhat*	*Not at all*
undertake a search of the literature?	*Very*	*Somewhat*	*Not at all*
find readily available evidence?	*Very*	*Somewhat*	*Not at all*
weigh up available evidence?	*Very*	*Somewhat*	*Not at all*
decide if changes in practice are warranted?	*Very*	*Somewhat*	*Not at all*
make changes in practice as appropriate?	*Very*	*Somewhat*	*Not at all*

2 Have you ever searched the literature yourself for an answer to a question?   *Yes / No*

If 'Yes':

▶ which database(s) have you used?

Medline   Cochrane   Internet   Other (what?)

▶ where did you search the literature?

Medical library   At work   At home   Other (where?)

▶ did you have any help in searching the literature?

None   Medical librarian   Friend/family   Work colleague   Other (who?)

3 Have you ever asked someone else to search the literature for you?   *Yes / No*

If 'Yes':

▶ who did the search for you?

▶ why didn't you do the search yourself?

*Lack of time   Lack of skill   Lack of access   Other reason
to databases*

4 Can you complete the following list from your own knowledge, describing the features of different types or levels of evidence in decreasing order of robustness from very strong evidence to none at all?

Type	Features
I	Strong evidence from at least one systematic review of multiple, well-designed, randomized controlled trials
II	
III	
IV	
V	
VI	No evidence at all

5 If you have previously searched for the evidence to answer a question you had posed, what did you do with the result of your search? (Circle all that apply.)

Discussed it with colleagues at work

Discussed it with friends or family

Made change(s) to an aspect of work

Decided against making any change(s) to any aspect of work

Other outcome – what?

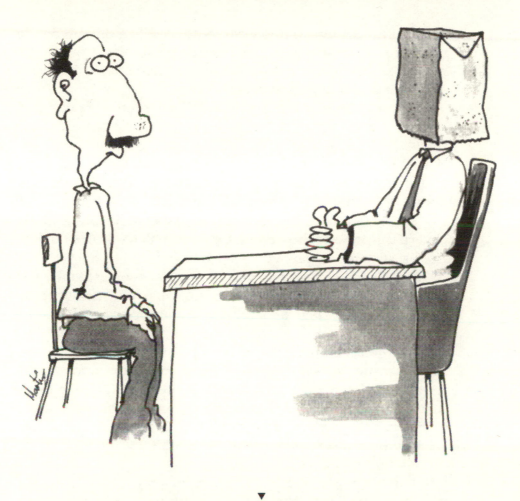

▼

Find out how to practise clinical effectiveness – don't shut your eyes to the changes going on around you.

What are clinical effectiveness and evidence-based health care?

Clinical effectiveness is 'the extent to which specific clinical interventions, when deployed in the field for a particular patient or population, do what they are intended to do – i.e. maintain and improve health and secure the greatest possible health gain from the available resources. To be reasonably certain that an intervention has produced health benefits, it needs to be shown to be capable of producing worthwhile benefit (efficacy and cost-effectiveness) and that it has produced that benefit in practice'.[1]

Evidence-based health care 'takes place when decisions that affect the care of patients are taken with due weight accorded to all valid, relevant information'.[2]

Evidence-based medicine is the 'conscientious, explicit, and judicious use of current best evidence in making decisions about the care of individual patients. The practice of evidence-based medicine means integrating individual clinical expertise with the best available external clinical evidence from systematic research'.[3]

A problem-solving approach based upon good evidence can also be applied to non-clinical decision making, such as most areas of management and resource allocation, as well as to clinical situations.

The three components of best possible clinical decision making[4,5] are *clinical expertise, patient preferences* and *clinical research evidence*. Clinical expertise and patient preferences may override the research evidence in some situations and for some patients. For example, patients may opt for less invasive treatment, or a sick patient may be too frail to undergo treatment with significant side-effects.

Clinical audit remains an important tool for determining whether actual performance compares with evidence-based standards and, if not, what changes are needed to improve performance. Clinical audit is 'the systematic and critical analysis of the quality of clinical care, including the procedures used for diagnosis, treatment and care, the associated use of resources and the resulting outcome and quality of life for the patient'.[1] In other words, clinical audit helps you to reach a standard of clinical work as near to best practice as possible.

The process of achieving evidence-based medicine can be divided into four sections:

1 the composition of a good question

2 a search of the literature to find the 'best' evidence available

3 an evaluation of what seems to be the most appropriate and relevant literature

4 the application of the evidence or findings.

What is the evidence for evidence-based health care?

There is growing evidence for the implementation of evidence-based health care.[6] Promoting Action on Clinical Effectiveness (PACE), a King's Fund programme, is developing evidence-based practice as a routine way of working for health services. An interim report[6] has described the successful outcomes when clinical effectiveness is linked to local needs and priorities so long as clinicians, managers, policy makers and patients are all involved in the process.

Practising in an evidence-based way:

▶ will promote your job satisfaction and feeling of being in control over your work

▶ can be used to justify maintaining or increasing budget allocations to particular areas of work

▶ will enhance your capability to do what's best for the patient.[7]

Why health professionals need information

Health professionals need to be well informed to be able to advise and inform patients appropriately. Patients who access the Internet and other electronic databases are starting to use that information to challenge clinicians' decisions about their care.

Clinicians will come under more pressure to respond to patients who have easy access to detailed information obtained from various sources, some of which will be inaccurate and misleading. The movement to patient empowerment has been generally welcomed, but may be threatening for clinicians who are insufficiently prepared to talk to well-informed patients, because they are unsure of their own knowledge base, time pressured, or do not understand how to assess what is the best evidence. The Royal College of General Practitioners has welcomed the evolving culture of patients' empowerment by access to information via the Internet, whilst at the same time expressing their concerns about how general practitioners will handle patients who are so knowledgeable about rare medical conditions.

Clinicians will need to develop skills in finding and judging medical information, and communicating such information to patients appropriately. Health professionals may lay themselves open to complaints or legal procedures if they fail to adopt best practice through ignorance of the available evidence. Clinicians need good communication skills as well as reliable information when advising patients.

In the future, patients will be increasingly encouraged to seek out information from the Internet themselves. Health professionals can help patients by indicating which electronic sources are most likely to be appropriate and reliable.

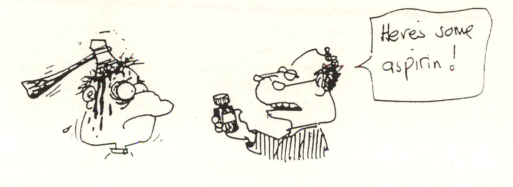

Quality of care may be compromised ...

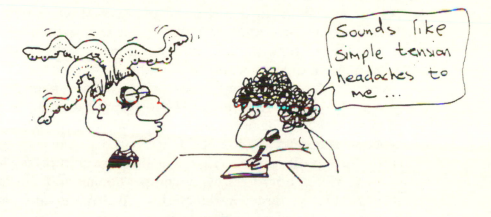

... without clinical effectiveness.

Are clinicians ready for evidence-based health care?

Recent surveys of general practitioners' perceptions of evidence-based medicine[7,8] found that GPs knew little about extracting information from journals, review publications and databases, and that few who were knowledgeable used these sources of information. Twenty per cent had access to bibliographic databases in their surgeries and 17% had access to the world wide web.[7] But the majority of GPs welcomed evidence-based medicine and agreed that it improves patient care.[7] GPs have been found to be more aware of publications that summarize evidence,[9] such as *Bandolier* and *Effective Health Care Bulletins*, rather than electronic databases; fundholding GPs were more likely than non-fundholding GPs to have referred to these publications. The researchers[7] concluded that the way forward in encouraging primary care clinicians to adopt evidence-based health care lay in promoting and improving access to summaries of evidence, and encouraging those primary care clinicians who are skilled in accessing and interpreting evidence to develop local evidence-based guidelines and advice.

One study[8] concluded that what was needed was a culture whereby health professionals posed 'regular questions about the validity of patient care' and developed 'skills both in defining useful questions and finding the answers'.

When GPs were asked what training they wanted in evidence-based practice, just over half wanted training in the use of the Medline database.[8]

Adverse comments about evidence-based practice include fear of the imposition of too rigid a health care culture, the loss of an overriding duty to provide compassionate and sensitive care[10] and that wholesale evidence-based practice is unrealistic because it is not affordable.[11] Some people mistrust the research–evidence base component of evidence-based practice because of the unreliability of some of the published literature; study biases are not always sufficiently recognized or acknowledged and, in occasional cases, have been discredited by sensational scandals involving researchers falsifying data.[12]

A needs assessment of multidisciplinary clinical staff working in acute Trusts in the West Midlands[13] discovered significant unease about the conversion from a clinical audit to a clinical effectiveness culture. Several practical difficulties constraining the uptake of evidence-based health care were a recurring theme: poor access to information and electronic databases, lack of understanding about the definition and advantages of evidence-based practices, and the widespread need for staff training in critical appraisal skills.

The Get Research Into Practice (GRIP) project in the West Midlands[14] has described many ways to accelerate the adoption of evidence-based practice and associated skills. The Aggressive Research Intelligence Facility (ARIF),[15] which is a collaboration between public health, epidemiology, general practice and health service management centres, exists to advance the use of evidence in the provision of health care in the West Midlands region. ARIF's regular reports describe the reviews and appraisals of the evidence the unit has provided in response to questions posed mainly by purchasers. The answers can be duplicated when others request the same information.

Learning by portfolio

Portfolio-based learning has been promoted since the early 1990s as a style of education that allows individuals to progress at their own pace. People can adopt education relevant to their needs, and composing a portfolio allows plenty of opportunities for reflection. Portfolio-based learning is not an easy option[16] compared to relatively passive types of learning such as listening to lectures. It takes a great deal of effort to complete a successful portfolio built on your past experiences and to progress through the stages of gathering and processing new information, critical reflection, interpretation and application. But it is worth it. The satisfaction that comes from completing a portfolio is as much about being in control of your own education as is acquiring new knowledge, attitudes and/or skills.[17,18]

Another advantage of composing a portfolio is that on-the-job learning is relevant to your work and life, and this is likely to retain your interest. At the end of the project you will have discovered that you have further educational and developmental needs. You will then have to decide whether or not you have taken learning about this topic, as to how to practise clinical effectiveness, as far as your resources permit (time, cost and effort).

So, using a portfolio-based approach to acquire the basic ability to practise clinical effectiveness, you should aim in this work programme to:

▸ identify the learning task(s), e.g. what capability you need to be able to practise clinical effectiveness
▸ set learning goals, e.g. learn to frame a question; search for, interpret and apply the evidence
▸ identify ways of achieving your goals by, for example, working through this book, peer group discussion, visiting colleagues, undertaking a (supervised) library search, exploring the Internet, reading more widely, making changes at work
▸ identify learning resources, e.g. the books and electronic databases in the medical library, the Internet, books, journals, video tuition tapes, local courses, correspondence from hospital specialists
▸ monitor how well the learning is going, e.g. reflect on the development of your knowledge and skills, seek a colleague's view of your work
▸ list your achievements, e.g. run through a cycle of clinical effectiveness
▸ use what you have learned, e.g. make change(s) at work as a result of obtaining evidence or new information as part of clinical governance.

Some people prefer to work alone, whilst others find that having a mentor to help build the portfolio is useful. A mentor can help to assess learning needs, develop a study plan, support and challenge the work done, identify further learning gaps, and generally help the person being mentored to stay on course. To some extent the way that this clinical effectiveness learning programme is set out obviates the need for a mentor, but if you think a mentor might facilitate your work, consider asking your local GP or Continuing Medical Education

(CME) tutor to act as a mentor; or maybe a colleague could work alongside you sharing the course too, as a 'co-mentor' or 'buddy'.[16]

Clinical effectiveness requires real commitment.

Electronic databases

The Internet

The Internet is the largest computer network in the world to which almost any type of computer can link. Most academic institutions are connected to the Joint Academic Network (JANET) and its Internet service (JIPS); staff and students can then access the Internet free on campus, or can dial up from home via a modem for the cost of a local phone call. Once an NHS-wide network is established there is the potential for NHS staff to have similar access to the Internet.

Information can be extracted from the Internet or exchanged via the world wide web (www) by electronic mail, telnet, newsgroups, network news, file transfer protocol and gopherspace (a system of interlinked menus which allows access to many Internet resources). The world wide web is a system for providing access to a network of interlinked documents and information services across the Internet. Documents can be stored on the web as text, images, sound or video. The language that the web clients and servers use to communicate with each other is called 'hypertext transfer protocol' (http).

To use the world wide web you need software called a *browser* (or *client*) to view www documents, such as *Netscape*. If you want to read more about searching the Internet, further details are given in the ABC of Medical Computing series.[19]

Various companies such as CompuServe and Microsoft Network offer on-line services. CompuServe provides access to shopping services, technical support, world news, and so on. CompuServe also links into the wider world of the Internet.

Medline

Medline is free to doctors who are BMA members – join by completing a form on the BMA's web site. Medline is available on CD-ROM or on-line via a PC (you will need a modem). It is produced by the National Library of Medicine in the United States. It contains about nine million references dating from 1966, drawn from 3600 journals in 70 countries, mainly those in *Index Medicus, Index to Dental Literature* and *International Nursing.* Abstracts are available for 70% of the entries.

There is free access to several health-related sites on Medline, amongst which are:

▶ HealthGate at http://www.healthgate.com/HealthGate/ MEDLINE/search.shtml
▶ Medscape at http://www.medscape.com/ (provides on-line articles about a wide range of medical specialties, plus a journal club).

The BMA library Medline Plus has added a new database, Embase, which concentrates on drug research and research carried out in Europe. It is more up to date than Medline. Members can access Medline Plus through the BMA pages on the Internet, or by direct access to the database. The new service is available at medline@bma.org.uk.

Cochrane library

http://www.cochrane.co.uk. 'This [the Cochrane library] is the single best source of reliable evidence about the effects of health care'.[20] The Cochrane library includes:

▶ The Cochrane Database of Systematic Reviews (CDSR). These are structured, systematic reviews of controlled trials. Evidence is included or excluded according to explicit quality criteria. A meta-analysis is undertaken by combining data from different studies to increase the *power* of the findings.
▶ The Database of Abstract of Reviews of Effectiveness (DARE). This is a database of research reviews of the effectiveness of health care interventions and the management and organization of health services. The reviews are

critically appraised by reviewers at the NHS Centre for Reviews and Dissemination at the University of York.

► The Cochrane Controlled Trials Register (CCTR). This bibliography of controlled trials has been compiled by hand searches through the world's literature. The Register includes reports from conference proceedings.

CINAHL

The Cumulative Index to Nursing and Allied Health Literature (CINAHL) is compiled by CINAHL Information Systems in the USA. It is a comprehensive database of 950 journals in the English language, relating to nursing and allied health disciplines covering such topics as health education, occupational therapy, and social services in health care.

Subject-specific bibliographic databases[21,22]

Some of those available on the Internet are:

► BIOETHICSLINE at http://www.healthgate.com/Health Gate/MEDLINE/search.shtml. This is a source of international bioethical literature from 1973 onwards, including newspaper articles, books and court judgements.

► PsycINFO at http://www.healthgate.com/HealthGate/price/b.psycinfo.html. This database includes worldwide literature from 1967 on psychology and psychological aspects of medicine.

Medical sites on the Internet[21,22]

▶ Health on the Net at http://www.hon.ch. The Health on the Net Foundation has developed a code of conduct for medical and health web sites. This states that medical information should either be given by medically trained and qualified professionals or, if this is not possible, it should be indicated clearly that the information is given by non-medically qualified people. Web sites complying with this code bear the Health on the Net logo. But the presence of a logo is not a guarantee of the quality of the information.

▶ Medical Matrix at http://www.medmatrix.org. This database is published by Healthtel links, with around 4000 quality-assessed Internet sites of clinical medicine topics ranked for quality.

▶ TRIP database at http://www.gwent.nhs.gov.uk/trip/ is a one-stop search engine for evidence-based material on the Internet. There are over 1100 searchable hyper-links including *Bandolier*, the Cochrane database and the *Evidence-Based Medicine* journal.

▶ Bath Information and Data Service (BIDS)[19] at http://www.bids.ac.uk is a database designed to be used by non-expert searchers and includes several medically orientated databases such as Embase, Citation Indexes, and Inside Information, with a wide variety of medically related reference material.

Web site for learning evidence-based medicine skills[23]

EBM at McMaster University at http://hiru.hirunet.mcmaster.ca/ebm/default.htm includes users' guides based on treatment and management of real cases.

Useful software

The Oxford Clinical Mentor[24] (OCM) is an electronic medical knowledge clinical support system developed by Oxford University Press with EMIS practice computer systems. It has information about more than 2000 diseases cross-referenced with about 25 000 commonly used medical terms. The programme comes up with a differential diagnosis for a set of symptoms, signs and test results, suggesting appropriate management plans which are a mix of evidence-based medicine and best practice. The information is regularly updated as new literature is published.

Electronic journals

All the titles listed below can be accessed free of charge. Some of the web sites show the full contents of the journal, others do not carry the full text of all original articles.

▶ *British Medical Journal*
http://www.bmj.com
▶ *The Lancet*
http://www.thelancet.com

> 'The greatest obstacle to discovering the truth is being convinced that you already know it.'

Asking the right question[25]

Although you may be burning to ask your question, when you actually try to set it down on paper, you may find that the exercise is more difficult than you think.

Questions have to be phrased in a very specific way to obtain meaningful responses in any context. This applies to asking other people what they think about a topic as much as for searching the literature for the best evidence.

The best clinical questions relate to queries arising from your own patients during the course of your work rather than being hypothetical questions. Relevant work-based questions should motivate you to seek the evidence and make change(s). Before you go to a lot of trouble to find answers or solutions to your questions, ask around at work and find out if anyone else is concerned about the same question or problem, already has the answer(s), or knows where to find them.

The question should be:

► simple
► specific
► realistic
► important
► capable of being answered
► agreed and owned by those who will be involved in any changes resulting
► implementable
► about a topic where change will be possible.

Think about how to construct your clinical question by considering:

► what the question is about. For example, is the question about an individual or group of patients? What are the patient characteristics you are interested in, such as age or gender? Is it a clinical dilemma or a resource problem?
► the setting. For example, is it specific to primary, secondary or community care, rural or urban locations?
► the type of intervention and whether it is being compared with current practice or another intervention. For example, are you interested in different treatments, causes, prognostic factors or risks, compared with current practice or no treatment?
► the outcome(s) of the clinical topic. For example, is an acceptable outcome to your question reduced numbers of cases of diseases, reduced patients' suffering, or increased quality of life?

You should focus and phrase your question to include whatever it is that you want to know about effects, efficiency, diagnosis or prognosis. You may decide to have a main question with several subsidiary questions.

Questions about cost-effectiveness

Cost-effectiveness is not synonymous with 'cheap'.

A cost-effective intervention is one which gives a better or equivalent benefit from the intervention in question for lower or equivalent cost, or where the relative improvement in outcome is higher than the relative difference in cost. In other words, being cost-effective means having the best outcomes for the least input. Using the term 'cost-effective' implies that you have considered potential alternatives.

An intervention must first be considered *clinically* effective to warrant investigation into its potential to be *cost*-effective. Evidence-based practice must incorporate clinical judgement. You have to interpret the evidence when it comes to applying

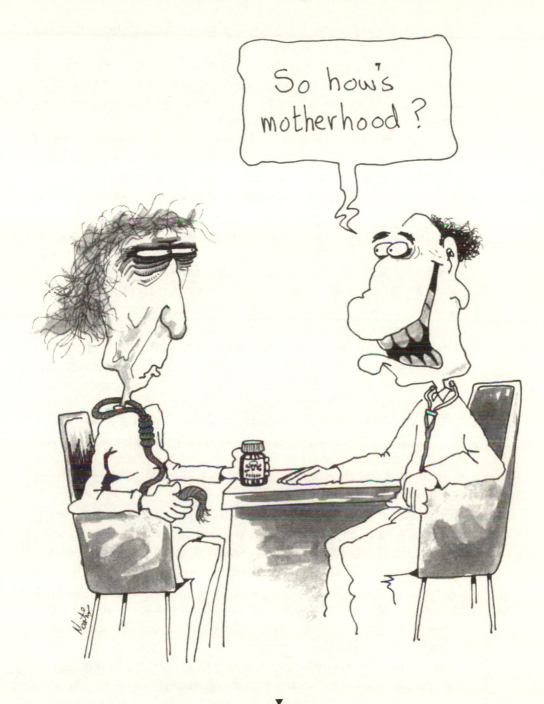

Asking inappropriate questions.

it to individual patients, whether it be evidence about clinical effectiveness or cost-effectiveness.

If you want to ask a question about cost-effectiveness you should be sure to have confirmed clinical effectiveness first, and have gone on to ask a question about cost-effectiveness as the second stage in seeking the evidence.

A 'benefit' is what is gained from meeting a chosen need and a 'cost' is the benefit that would have been obtained from using the same resources in an alternative way. Opportunity costs are the costs of the benefits foregone in deploying resources in the chosen way.

A new or alternative treatment or intervention should be compared directly with the next best treatment or intervention.

An economic evaluation is a comparative analysis of two or more alternatives in terms of their costs and consequences.[26] There are four different types: cost-effectiveness, cost minimization, cost–utility analysis and cost–benefit analysis. Cost-effectiveness analysis is used to compare the effectiveness of two interventions with the same treatment objectives. Cost minimization compares the costs of alternative treatments which have identical health outcomes. Cost–utility analysis enables the effects of alternative interventions to be measured against a combination of life expectancy and quality of life, a common outcome measure being 'quality-adjusted life-years' (QALYs). A cost–benefit analysis compares the incremental costs and benefits of a programme.

Efficiency is sometimes confused with effectiveness. Being efficient means having obtained the most quality from the least expenditure, or the required level of quality for the least expenditure. To measure efficiency you need to make a judgement about the level of quality of the 'purchase' and be able to relate it to 'price'. 'Price' alone does not measure efficiency. Quality is the indicator used in combination with price to assess whether something is more efficient.

So, cost-effectiveness is a measure of efficiency and suggests that costs have been related to effectiveness.

> 'I have finally made up my mind but the decision was by no means unanimous.'

Framing questions: some examples

Now try these two examples of clinical situations and frame a specific question for each with which you might search the literature for evidence to answer the question.

Jot down notes under each heading and write the final question at the bottom of the page ready to do a trial literature search using the Medline database. Refine and limit the question to what would seem to be a relevant question for those working in primary care. Your question should be shaped by thinking out exactly why you are asking it and how you might apply the evidence in practice once you have obtained it.

Set a question to address problem 1

A general practice is taking stock of the preventive work it does and is reviewing whether to continue the range of work that different health professionals offer. The staff are wondering what the impact is of the range of health education about smoking that they offer their patients.

1 What is the question about – an individual patient, a group of people, a particular population, patient characteristics, a clinical dilemma, a resource problem?

2 What is the setting or context of the clinical topic/situation?

3 Is there an intervention and, if so, with what is it being compared?

4 What is/are the outcome(s) of the clinical topic?

5 What is the specific question you will ask?

6 Choose up to four key words, in priority order, that you
   think best represent the important components of your
   question and restrict it as far as possible to your field of
   enquiry.

Some example details follow.

Example details of question posed to address problem 1

Defining the question

The refined question should narrow down the limits of
the enquiry by specifying as many of the following details as
apply:

▶ What is the question about – the whole or a section of the
  practice population? What is meant by health education?
  Which staff are involved with the health education
  intervention? What is meant by 'smoking', etc.?
▶ What is the setting or context of the enquiry? The focus of
  your interest might be general practice, the community or
  primary care; or a particular type of clinic in the practice.
▶ Is there an intervention and, if so, with what is it being
  compared? What types of health education is the questioner
  interested in? Is there any way of practise to which health
  education is being compared?

▶ What is/are the outcome(s) of the health education intervention and what is meant by 'impact'? e.g. changes in attitudes, knowledge of or quantity of cigarettes smoked; reduction in disease severity or frequency.

▶ The specific question will have narrowed down the problem to one in which the practice staff are interested. For instance, if the staff in the practice were reviewing whether to continue the teenage lifestyles clinic, besides looking at attendance figures, patient preferences, and opportunity costs for staff, the practice team might want to know 'what is the evidence for the effectiveness of giving adolescents face-to-face education about the risks of cigarette smoking in nurse-run clinics?' A more general question might be 'what is the evidence for the effectiveness of a health professional advising a smoker to stop smoking?'

▶ Key words might be *health education*, *smoking*, *primary health care*, *adolescents*, etc. depending on your question. You might have other key words.

Comments from participants' experiences at the live workshops on clinical effectiveness

Participants found that each small group composed entirely different questions as they had different foci of interests. Some found that their question did not contain the key words they selected after finalizing their question, as they had not refined their ideas sufficiently. The result was that in some cases a later search on the chosen key words on Medline missed the point of the question.

Set a question to address problem 2

A mother asks a health professional about her child's eczema and whether it is worth going to all the bother of trying to minimize the amount of house dust lying around at home.

Have a go at completing parts of the question for problem 2:

1 What is the question about – an individual patient, a group of people, a particular population, patient characteristics, a clinical dilemma, a resource problem?

2 What is the setting or context of the clinical topic/situation?

3 Is there an intervention and, if so, with what is it being compared?

4 What is/are the outcome(s) of the clinical topic?

5 What is the specific question you will ask?

6 Choose up to four key words in priority order that you think best represent the important components of your question and restrict them as far as possible to your field of enquiry.

Some example details follow.

Example details of question posed to address problem 2

Defining the question

A refined question will narrow down the limits of the enquiry by specifying as many of the following details as apply:

▸ What is the question about – the child or the practice population as a whole? What is meant by house dust – or house dust mite? What is meant by eczema? Is there any other condition that it would be more important to search on, e.g. asthma?

▸ What is the setting or context of the enquiry? The focus of your interest might be general practice, the community or primary care, or a particular age of house.

▸ If there is an intervention, with what is it being compared – the method of eradication of house dust, or any other type of intervention such as other treatments for eczema?

▸ What is/are the outcome(s) of the health education intervention and what is meant by *minimize* – changes in symptoms, reduction in frequency of flare-ups, etc.?

▸ The specific question should narrow down the problem to one in which the mother and health professional are interested. For instance, to be able to apply her new knowledge, the mother will want to know the best method to use if the health professional advises that minimizing house dust is effective. So you might ask 'what is the evidence for the effectiveness of measures to minimize the quantity of house dust mites on the severity of eczema?'

▸ Key words might be *allergy, dermatitis, eczema, mites, dust*. You might have other key words.

Examples of questions posed by the participants of the clinical effectiveness workshops

These are not given as examples that show particularly good or bad question formats, they are included here to show the range and variety of questions that individual participants in the workshops developed in conjunction with others in their practice or health care setting. These are the questions they used to search for the evidence, and when they found evidence, to interpret it and decide whether or not to put that evidence into practice.

- Is it cost-effective to screen all diabetics for microalbuminuria?
- Is the routine use of potassium-sparing diuretics in association with loop diuretics clinically justifiable?
- How effective is involving health-care support workers (as opposed to qualified nursing staff) in continence reviews?
- Is there any evidence that a vegetarian diet reduces the incidence of bowel cancer?
- Do raised triglyceride levels have an adverse effect on diabetics? If so, what treatment is advised?
- Is an optimal outcome for patients with breast cancer treated by lumpectomy dependent on follow-up in a secondary care clinic?
- Are there any dangers in using mouthwashes?
- Is there a link between a history of potential tooth decay and the possibility of decay in children's teeth?
- Should maintenance doses of thyroxine be given in accordance with blood levels of thyroxine or the presence of patients' symptoms?
- Do practice registers of patients with coronary heart disease improve patient care?
- Has any work been published on integrated care pathways in leukaemia?
- What is the outcome of patients developing pneumonia who have had pneumonia vaccine over the past five years?
- Are head lice best treated by malathion or permethrin?

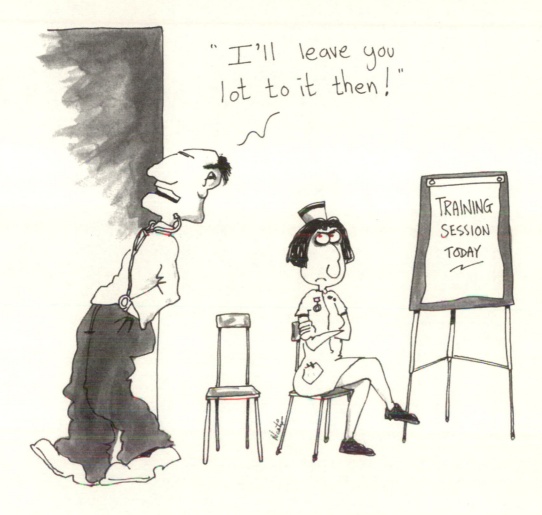

Clinical effectiveness is done best by involving the whole team.

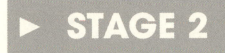

Undertaking a library search

The search strategy: think, search and appraise

A search for the best evidence follows the sequence of 'think, search and appraise'. This search strategy comprises:

- ▶ thinking about and defining a good specific question in consultation with all the staff who are involved in the question and affected by possible change(s)
- ▶ searching for and finding the best level of evidence by looking critically at the relevant publications obtained
- ▶ appraising and interpreting the evidence as applied to your question in relation to your situation.

Clinical effectiveness encompasses the whole cycle:

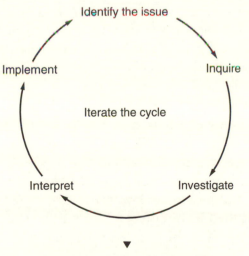

The clinical effectiveness cycle.

It is tempting for health professionals who are rushed for time and hot on the scent of evidence to a question to jump straight from an idea to carrying out a search, instead of working through the steps with the necessary rigour. Cutting corners wastes time in the long run if you ask the wrong question, answer a different question to the one you intended, or become distracted by lots of interesting but irrelevant literature.

How long you spend and to what lengths you go with a search will depend on its purpose. If you were commissioned to undertake a major systematic review, you would spend many months searching every relevant database, hand searching through papers and journals, hunting up conference proceedings, trying personal contacts, translating non-English language papers, and generally leaving no stone unturned in the pursuit of published and unpublished studies. But as you are probably a busy clinician who just wants to find the best evidence for answering a question in practice, you should strictly limit your search as your resources are limited. You will probably be better off spending your precious time doing several searches for different topics than doing one exhaustive search on a single subject. So stop your search as soon as you find a relevant systematic review of multiple, well-designed, randomized controlled trials in the Cochrane database. If there is no such systematic review in the Cochrane database move on to look for a review in the Database of Abstracts of Effectiveness Reviews (DARE). If no luck there try Medline, or Embase or other specialist databases until you obtain the best possible level of evidence that you can find.

If you have not undertaken a search of the literature before you would be well advised to book an individual session with your local medical librarian and to undertake a search in your postgraduate medical library if this is possible. You should be able to teach yourself from guidebooks, these notes, and trial and error, but a medical librarian is the person with the know-how about the best medical terms and phrases to try with your search. You as a health professional will know about the validity, context and relevance of search words and phrases as applied to your question. Together, you as a clinician and the medical librarian make a strong search team.

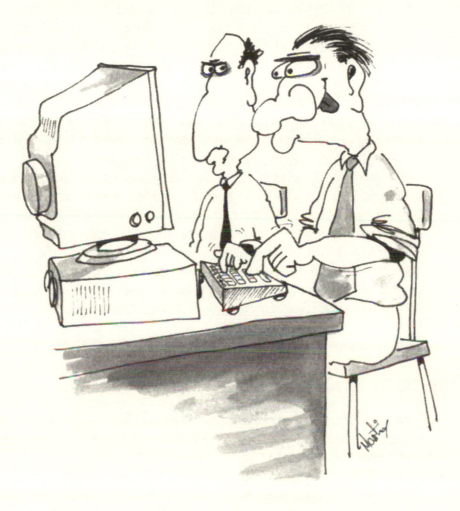

▼

Book up with a medical librarian to help you search.

Undertake a search

Before you start *write down* the key words you want to use and prioritize their order of importance. How many key words you enter as the first stage depends on how wide you expect your field of enquiry to be. If you key in *asthma* you would expect to identify thousands more references to published papers than if you keyed in the name of a rare condition. So if you are searching within a broad topic area such as *asthma* you should prepare more potential words to narrow the field of your search for the few most relevant papers that will supply evidence to answer your original question. Refine your question prior to your search so that it is very focused and make sure that the key words are the most pertinent you can manage. Then you will spend less time on your search and have more chance of finding the most appropriate published evidence. So if you want to know more in the subject area of *asthma*, build your question carefully. Aim specifically at the purpose of the question and include the setting, the population under question, the intervention, the outcome and any other important details.

Using the Cochrane database

Enter your most important key words first – perhaps two words, as there are relatively few publications on the Cochrane database compared to other databases. Look at the different levels of evidence from the systematic reviews on the Cochrane Database of Systematic Reviews (CDSR) to controlled trials on the Cochrane Controlled Trials Register (CCTR) to the abstracts on the Database of Abstracts of Reviews of Effectiveness (DARE). The hierarchy of evidence is explained further in the next section.

It is likely that you will obtain only a small number of references to relevant-sounding systematic reviews because, as mentioned above, the Cochrane has relatively few publications on its databases in comparison to others. It is more likely that you will not find a relevant systematic review, but will identify many references to controlled trials. You should then modify your search further by entering the first two key words again plus a third key word that was your next choice in priority order in your original list of key words constructed prior to beginning your search. If this has not refined your search enough, repeat the exercise, adding a fourth key word. When you have narrowed your search sufficiently, print off the abstracts of the papers you have identified and obtain copies of the original articles as appropriate so that you can critically appraise them yourself.

Do not assume that the contents of any paper published in a journal are valid, reliable or accurate, however reputable the journal. Mistakes may have been overlooked, studies reported might not be relevant to your own situation, or the results may not be generalizable to your question.

If your search on the Cochrane database has been unsuccessful, move on to another database which has many more references to medical publications, such as Medline.

Using the Medline database

Because Medline has a phenomenal number of references you will have to develop a very strict search strategy to narrow down your focus of enquiry. To operate a search on Medline, you can use the key words that occur in its thesaurus of medical terms, the medical subject heading list (MeSH). There are over 17 500 MeSH terms arranged as a tree structure with broad subject areas branching off and sub-dividing into narrower subject terms. If you key in a word which is not a MeSH term, Medline will give you a choice of terms with close meanings. For instance if you key in 'primary care', which is not a key word in MeSH, Medline offers you 'primary health care', amongst others; if you key in 'cigarettes', which is not a key word in MeSH, Medline will give you 'smoking', 'smoking cessation' or 'cannabis smoking' as alternative words or phrases.

You can trace published literature on Medline by either searching for your own key word(s) in the title, abstract, author's name, or body of any articles or papers, or by searching for articles containing selected words from the MeSH list.

Entering one key word will often yield thousands of references to published articles. So, you can do a more selective search by combining key words using the instructions 'and' and 'or' (these are called Boolean operators). To narrow the search further you can restrict the numbers of years of literature searched, the language the paper is written in, the papers in the journals of the abridged *Index Medicus*, and specify 'human' as opposed to 'animal' research.

In a medical library, all you will need to do to access Medline or the Cochrane databases is to click on the icons on your screen, signposting you to the relevant databases. You may use Ovid software or another standard communications programme to access the Medline service.

There are two publications which give easy-to-follow practical details of undertaking a Medline search[27,28] which you could consult if you are unfamiliar with Medline searching and want to read more about the process before having a go for yourself.

Hints for the use of Medline (adapted from Ovid Technologies software) are:

▶ click on a **Subject Heading** to view its tree of key words or terms
▶ select the **Explode** box to retrieve references using your selected key word and all the more specific terms stemming from it
▶ select the **Focus** box to limit your search to those documents in which your key word (subject heading) is considered to be the main point of the article
▶ if the topic of your search does not map to a desirable subject heading, click on the box **Search as Keyword**.

You will learn most by having a go. You really cannot do anything wrong that you are not able to put right by retracing your steps. There are help boxes and icons throughout the database forms.

The hierarchy of evidence

The table below shows the generally agreed strengths of evidence ranging from level I, which is the most robust evidence, to level V based on the opinions of experts in the field.[25] But there may not be any evidence in the literature for answering the question(s) you are posing.

Type	Evidence
I	Strong evidence from at least one systematic review of multiple, well-designed, randomized controlled trials
II	Strong evidence from at least one properly designed, randomized controlled trial of appropriate size
III	Evidence from well-designed trials without randomization, single group pre–post, cohort, time series or matched case–control studies
IV	Evidence from well-designed non-experimental studies from more than one centre or research group
V	Opinions of respected authorities, based on clinical evidence, descriptive studies or reports of expert committees

The most valid types of research for extracting evidence about clinical effectiveness are randomized controlled trials, followed by controlled trials, then trials and, less reliably, observational studies. A systematic review of several randomized controlled studies or all known studies is better than a review of some studies, which in turn is better than a report of a case study. You should start to search for the best evidence and, if you do not find it, work down the hierarchy.

If there is no reliable evidence to be found after searching the Cochrane, Medline and other relevant databases, you should then move on to look for any expert consensus agreements by multidisciplinary groups.

Be realistic – try and find one or a few key reviews rather than get bogged down in a plethora of papers. Clinical effectiveness is a tool for keeping up to date with your clinical practice, retaining your professional interest and enhancing your effectiveness – spending too much time pursuing it may be counterproductive.

> 'Most of my problems either have no answer or else the answer is worse than the problem.'

Examples

Example of literature search using problem 1 described previously

Question: What is the evidence for the effectiveness of a health professional advising a smoker to stop smoking?

Key words: *health education, smoking, primary health care, family practice*

Selected Medline database <1995 to April 1998>

The search used the MeSH words *health education, smoking, primary health care, family practice* fed in one at a time to build up the search.

Set	Search	Results
1	explode *health education/*	8107
2	explode *smoking/*	7803
3	(combine) 1 and 2	341
4	limit 3 to English language	299
5	explode *primary health care/*	4290
6	*family practice/*	5462
7	(combine) 5 or 6	9292
8	(combine) 4 and 7	17

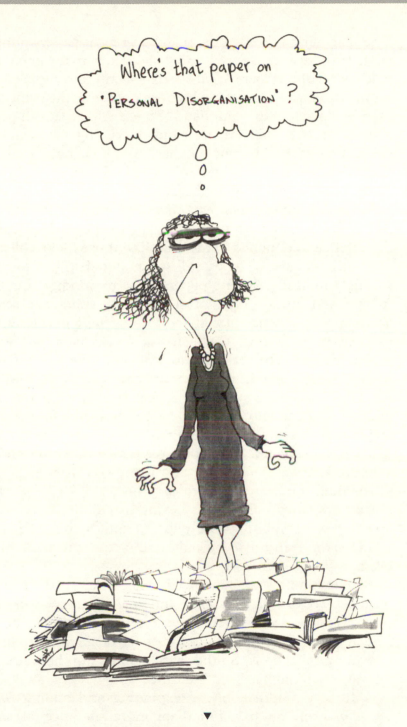

Use IT to ask a question and search for the evidence systematically.

The searcher has limited the search to recent papers published from 1995 onwards. Sets 1 and 2 show how many papers were held by Medline where *health education* and *smoking* were listed on the database. Someone who does not know the subject field very well may use the command 'explode' to access all possible articles on the database, to avoid restricting the search to a subsection of the Medline database 'tree'. Using the 'explode' function avoids relying on the MeSH indexer, with whose categorization you may not agree.

Set 3 combines *health education* and *smoking* to find those 341 papers where both these key words appear. Set 4 confines the references obtained in the search to those 299 publications written in English. This is still too many abstracts to browse through to find relevant papers. So, to modify the search further and focus on the most relevant papers, the searcher added *primary health care* in set 5 and *family practice* in set 6 to specify the setting in which *health education* and *smoking* was of interest. The search word *primary health care* has several branches and that is why the searcher has 'exploded' it in set 5 so that none of the branches are missed; but *family practice* is at the end of a branch and has therefore not been 'exploded'. The reason that both *primary health care* and *family practice* were included was that papers from inside and out-side the UK were of interest and many countries such as the USA might be more likely to use the term *family practice* in place of *primary health care*. Keying in *primary health care* or *family practice* found 9292 papers, and many publications would have been missed if only one of these terms had been used.

By combining sets 4 and 7 (that is, looking for papers that have key words *health education* and *smoking* and *primary health care* or *family practice*), references were found to 17 papers. It is realistic to scroll through this number of abstracts to look for relevant publications. So the search could stop here if enough relevant material has been identified.

A further modification by exploding and adding *smoking cessation* would not have found any more references as *smoking cessation* is a branch of *smoking*.

A search may be narrowed further by introducing the word 'not' and by linking adjacent words that might equally well stand alone.[27]

An experienced medical librarian is an invaluable guide for a novice searcher. Besides knowing alternative terms such as *family practice* and *primary health care* as already described, the librarian will be aware of what words may be spelt differently by researchers in different countries, likely categories for your subject areas, and which databases are most appropriate for the topic of your search.

Example of literature search using problem 2 described previously

Question: What is the evidence for the effectiveness of measures to minimize the quantity of house dust mites on the severity of eczema?

Key words: *allergy, dermatitis, eczema, mites, dust*

Cochrane database

If the advanced search option is tried, using one of the key words *eczema* or *dermatitis* and, in addition, *mite** (using the * after mite means that if mite is only a part of the word included in the database the reference will still appear), 206 references are identified for *mite**, 602 with the key word *dermatitis*, and 271 for *eczema*. Using a combination of *dermatitis* or *eczema*, 753 'hits' are scored; adding *mite** at this point gains 17 'hits' – no systematic reviews (CSDR), no abstracts of reviews (DARE), and 17 references to controlled trials (CCTR), of which two seem appropriate:

▶ Tan BB, Weald D, Strickland I, Friedmann PS (1996) Double-blind controlled trial of effect of house-dust mite allergen avoidance on atopic dermatitis. *Lancet.* **347**: 15–18.

▶ Hide DW, Matthews S, Matthews L *et al.* (1994) Effect of allergen avoidance in infancy on allergic manifestations at age two years. *J Allergy Clin Immunol.* **93**: 842–6.

A 'belt and braces' technique makes sure you do not miss anything and you might key in '*dust.tx*' instead. This identifies any article on the database where *dust* is a textword (*tx*) that appears in the abstract. This reduces your reliance on the Cochrane indexer and minimizes your chances of missing any paper relating to *house dust* that an indexer has categorized differently to the way in which you would have expected.

Medline database

Selected Medline database <1995 to April 1998>

Set	Search	Results
1	explode *eczema/*	296
2	explode *dermatitis/*	4730
3	(alternative)1 or 2	4730
4	explode *mites/*	766
5	(combine) 3 and 4	67
6	*dust/*	925
7	*dust.tw*	1594
8	6 or 7	1805
9	5 and 8	37
10	limit 9 to English language	31

Exploding the key words *dermatitis* and *eczema* in sets 1 and 2 and then combining them in set 3 ensures that all papers are identified where either the word *eczema* or *dermatitis* is used. Take care about keying in 'and' and 'or'. Keying in '1 and 2' in set 3 would have meant that identified articles must contain both of those words, which was obviously not the intention of the search.

Modifying the search in set 5 by adding *mites* found 67 papers. Adding *dust* modified the search further so that by set

10 there were 31 papers. The searcher did not explode *dust* on this occasion, because *dust* is one of the MeSH words in the Medline database, with many irrelevant branches such as *cosmic dust* which, if followed, would identify similarly irrelevant papers. The searcher had already noted that *dust* on Medline included *house dust* as a branch. To reduce the chances of missing any relevant papers, the searcher used the textword abbreviated as *dust.tw* to identify an extra 669 papers (1594–925) where *dust* appeared anywhere in the text on the database but had not been classified as a MeSH word by the Medline cataloguer.

Browsing through the 31 abstracts on the screen found six that looked interesting. One of these seemed very relevant to the question:

▶ Tan BB, Weald D, Strickland I, Friedmann PS (1996) Double-blind controlled trial of effect of house-dust mite allergen avoidance on atopic dermatitis. *Lancet*. **347**: 15–18.

This is an example of a search strategy that has been designed not to miss any papers by starting out to look as widely as possible for references and then gradually narrowing down the search. If the searcher had keyed in the instruction to *focus* on 'dust', this might have been exclusive.

It is a good idea to print out the results of your search before you leave the screen, making concurrent notes on the paper print-out to remind you of the stages of your search, otherwise it will be a meaningless jumble at the end.

Example of search using one of the workshop participant's questions

Question: Is it cost-effective to screen all diabetics for micro-albuminuria?

Key words: *microalbuminuria, diabetes mellitus, screening, cost-effectiveness*

Cochrane database

Keying in the umbrella term *diabet** ensured that papers with the words *diabetic, diabetes, different types of diabetes* were all included.

Similarly the key word *microalbumin** ensured that words with slightly different endings were all included. Browsing through the MeSH headings for *diabet** in the Cochrane database reveals many specific types of diabetes in the thesaurus; exploding *diabet** identifies more than 2900 references. Keying in *diabet** found 4132 references, whilst *diabetes* found 3479 references.

There was a total of 138 'hits' from searching on *microalbumin** and *diabet** in the Cochrane database. Three were 'hits' on the Cochrane Database of Systematic Reviews (CDSR), of which one was a complete review entitled 'Protein restriction in diabetic renal disease' which did not seem relevant to the question and two were protocols of reviews. There were references to 134 controlled trials in the Cochrane Controlled Trials Register (CCTR) and one 'hit' on the Database of Abstracts of Reviews of Effectiveness (DARE).

Modifying the search by adding the term *screen** reduced the number of controlled trials to six with one protocol featured in the CDSR.

As none of these articles seemed relevant, other search terms were added as *cost-effectiv** and *diabet**. This resulted in identifying 16 'hits' on the CDSR, 13 of which were complete reviews, plus 17 abstracts on the DARE, five controlled trials on the CCTR and four 'hits' on the Cochrane Collaboration of Collaborative Review Groups. None of these 'hits' were relevant to the question when the searcher browsed through the titles of the papers, so the searcher moved on to the Medline database.

Medline search

The word *microalbuminuria* did not exist in the MeSH index – *albuminuria* was the nearest match. Keying in *diabetes* gave a selection of search words in the McSH index under the umbrella term *diabetes* of *diabetes insulin dependent, diabetic neuropathies, hypertension, diabetes mellitus, cardiovascular diseases, risk factors, blood pressure, diabetic angiopathies, urinary tract infections;* the searcher chose to select *diabetes mellitus.* Keying in the word *screening* gave a choice of *mass screening, substance-related disorders, breast screening, cerebral aneurysm, diabetic retinopathy, colonoscopy, chlamydia trachomatis, neisseria gonorrhoea, sensitivity and specificity, colorectal neoplasm, diagnostic services* and *preventive health services.*

The table below describes the results of the search on Medline for evidence to answer the same question:

Set	Search	Results
1	*albuminuria/*	995
2	explode *diabetes mellitus/*	16 950
3	1 and 2	669
4	explode *mass screening/*	7721
5	*screen$.tw*	26 391
6	explode *preventive health services/*	16 449
7	4 or 5 or 6	38 199
8	3 and 7	48
9	limit 8 to English language	44

The search might be narrowed further by adding another modification, 'aim', which stands for 'Abridged *Index Medicus*', but these are mainly American journals and by doing this, you might miss UK-based publications.

This search demonstrates a strategy nicknamed 'building a hedge'. This will capture any references categorized under *mass screening, preventive health services* or *screening,* to cover all categories that the indexer might have selected according to MeSH headings. The term *screen$* is the equivalent way of displaying terms on Medline as *screen** is on the Cochrane database, to cover all key words starting with *screen.*

The great care necessary to avoid missing relevant publications is illustrated by the following paper not being categorized under *screening* in the MeSH categories despite it having this word in its title:

▸ Kiberd BA, Jindal KK (1995) Screening to prevent renal failure in insulin-dependent diabetic patients: an economic evaluation. *BMJ*. **311**: 1595–9.

The paper was actually inconclusive because the study population was limited to insulin-dependent diabetes and so it did not answer the question. But the only way it was identified was by the searcher setting up the instruction to search for all abstracts containing the key word *screen$.tw.*

Coincidentally, the medical librarian helping with this search remembered seeing a relevant paper in the local area's postgraduate journal:

▸ Davies S (1997) Microalbuminuria. *Midlands Medicine*. **20**: 67–9.

This was a very helpful paper which was not held on either of the Cochrane or Medline databases searched, being part of the 'grey' literature. It was consistent with level V in the hierarchy of evidence, describing the opinion of a local well-informed expert who stated that 'microalbuminuria has been identified as the strongest predictor of diabetic nephropathy, with 80–90% of affected patients going on to develop this problem' and recommended annual screening of diabetics aged 12–70 years for microalbuminuria. This article cited four other relevant references, three of which were published before 1995, and had therefore been missed in this Medline search which had been limited to published papers from 1995 onwards.

Another useful way of limiting a search is to see if your searching facilities permit you to confine your search to 'local holdings' of literature so that you can easily refer to original papers once you have identified the references from your computerized search.

As a result of the evidence gained from the search, the workshop participant who posed this question instituted routine testing of diabetics for microalbuminuria in the practices' protocols.

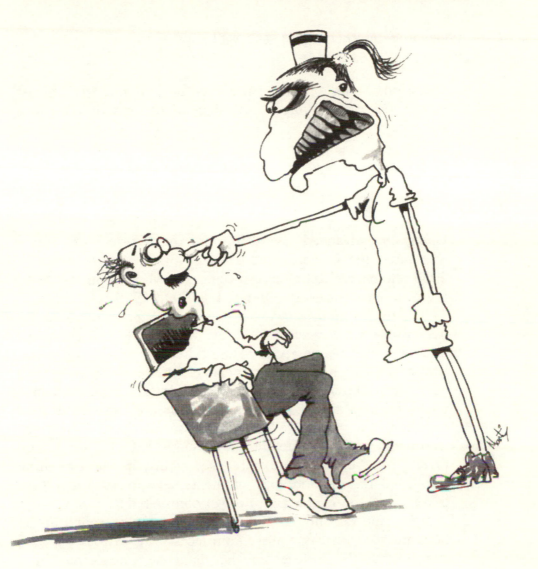

▼
Information is power!

Example of search using a second workshop participant's question

Question: Is an optimal outcome for patients with breast cancer treated by lumpectomy dependent on follow-up in a secondary care clinic?

Key words: *breast cancer, lumpectomy, follow-up*

Cochrane database

Using the 'advanced search' option, the phrase *breast cancer* was automatically converted to *breast and cancer* and revealed 2050 references. To be more specific, the MeSH option offered the term *breast neoplasms*, which identified 1895 references.

Adding 'or' *lumpectomy* to *breast and cancer* revealed six irrelevant-sounding systematic reviews (CDSR), 11 protocols and nine quality-assessed reviews on DARE (of which one was 'Improving outcomes in breast cancer: the research evidence') and 1952 references to controlled trials (CCTR). If such a paper covered the material you sought and answered your question you might well stop your search here. The term 'protocol' refers to the stage of development of a systematic review on the Cochrane database, when the authors have published the methodology of the review and the inclusion criteria and so on, but have not yet completed it.

It is important not to narrow your search too much at the beginning to restrict yourself unnecessarily or risk missing papers that the indexer of the database categorized in a different way from that which you would have expected.

As little appropriate information had been obtained from the search and the abstracts obtained did not appear to address the question of follow-up in primary or secondary care specifically, *follow** was keyed in, to produce a total of 883 'hits' on the Cochrane database. The searcher narrowed the focus further by adding in *general practice;* this key word was chosen as opposed to *primary care* or *secondary care* to avoid misinterpretation as meaning primary or secondary cancer in this instance. This modification achieved 51 'hits' on the Cochrane database and narrowed the output down to 26 controlled trials.

Browsing through the 51 references found one protocol that appeared useful:

▶ Fossati R (1998) Follow-up strategies in early breast cancer (Cochrane review). In: *Cochrane Library Issue 3*. Oxford Update Software, Oxford.

Medline database

Keying in *breast cancer* gave a choice of *breast neoplasm/mass screening/mammography/adenocarcinoma/proteins/antineoplastic agents, hormonal/case-control studies/age factors/antineoplastic agents, combined/tamoxifen. Lumpectomy* was not a word recognized in Medline; the options given were *mastectomy* or *mastectomy, segmental,* and the latter was chosen.

The search word *follow-up* resulted in a choice of *follow-up studies/coronary disease/laryngeal nerves/cornea/depressive disorder/ aged 80 or over/aging/factor viii/treatment outcome/myopia,* from which *follow-up studies* seemed the most pertinent.

The final choice of search words for the Medline database in the order intended to be tried were *breast neoplasm; mastectomy, segmental; follow-up studies.*

Set	Search	Results
1	explode *breast neoplasm/*	14 780
2	*mastectomy, segmental/*	433
3	1 or 2	14 795
4	*follow-up studies*	37 851
5	3 and 4	830
6	limit 5 to English language	717
7	*family practice/*	5462
8	explode *primary health care/*	4290
9	7 or 8	9292
10	6 and 9	11

Once the three chosen search terms had been keyed in and the 830 references resulting restricted to those in English language in set 6, the search was focused on the secondary care setting in line with the original question. However, keying in *secondary care* gave a selection of branch terms in the MeSH headings of which *family practice* and then *health services research* were the most popular options. The option *family practice* was selected as being the real setting of interest despite the original wording of the question, and the term *primary health care* was included too to reduce the chances of missing relevant papers. This identified 11 references in set 10. Browsing through the abstracts found two references of particular interest:

▶ Grunfeld E, Mant D, Vessey MP, Yudkin P (1995) Evaluating primary care follow-up of breast cancer: methods and preliminary results of three studies. *Annals of Oncology*. **6**: 47–52.
▶ Worster A, Wood ML, McWhinney IR, Bass MJ (1995) Who provides follow-up care for patients with early breast cancer? *Canadian Family Physician*. **41**: 1314–20.

Another way of tracking references and trying to make sure you are not missing any relevant ones, or opening a new avenue if you are stuck in your search down a blind alley, is to look down the list of references given in a relevant published paper to give you new ideas about which other MeSH headings you might explore.

In this case the searcher was aware of a paper published by Grunfeld *et al.* in 1996 that the search demonstrated here had failed to identify. The reason for the omission turned out to be that the term was written as *follow up* without a hyphen in the title of the 1996 paper (Grunfeld E, Mant D, Yudkin P, *et al.* (1996) Routine follow up of breast cancer in primary care: randomised trial. *BMJ*. **313**: 665–9) whereas the term *follow-up* in the MeSH heading had a hyphen. Searching on *follow up* without a hyphen identified the reference; the two Grunfeld *et al.* papers of 1995 and 1996 were indexed differently.

Searching by yourself

Now you do it – work through an example by yourself.

1 Take any one (or all) of the four problems which interests you most – whether health education on smoking is worth doing, the problem of the mother wanting to know if the likely improvement to her child's eczema warrants the efforts involved in minimizing house dust at home, whether it is cost-effective to screen all diabetics for microalbuminuria, or if patients who have had a lumpectomy for breast cancer are best followed up in secondary care. Adapt the problem(s) to your own circumstances. The idea of this exercise is that you will run a search on a similar question (or questions) to the ones already described so that you can follow the procedures laid out in this book for guidance, but adapted to your own situation so that it is more relevant to you. Conducting your own version of the search will give you more confidence that you can do a literature search yourself. Write in your own words what your perspective of the problem is:

2 Frame the words of your question to address that problem – the words you use in the question should vary from any presented in this book as the angle of the problem and the focus of the question should relate to your own circumstances. Write in your own words what the question is:

3 Choose up to five key words and put them in order of priority:

4 Undertake a search for the evidence to answer that problem. If possible go to your medical library and book time with a medical librarian and the computerized search facilities there. If the library has Cochrane and Medline searching facilities, use the Cochrane database first and then Medline.

Photocopy pages 51–4 if you undertake this exercise for more than one example question.

Cochrane search

▶ Write down how you will use your key words to search the Cochrane database. Which one, two or three words will you key in first? Then, which words will you add, and in what order, to narrow the focus of your search?

▶ How did the search go? How many 'hits' did you obtain from the Cochrane database?
  – systematic reviews on the Cochrane Database of Systematic Reviews (CDSR):
      (i) number of reviews =
      (ii) number of protocols =
  – controlled trials on the Cochrane Controlled Trials Register (CCTR) =
  – abstracts on the Database of Abstracts of Reviews of Effectiveness (DARE) =

▶ Write down up to five sets of details of articles that seem relevant to your question, giving article titles, authors' names, year of publication, volume of journal/source and page details so that you can obtain the original papers if you should wish to. Print off the abstracts if you have the facilities to do so.

Medline search

► Write down how you will use your key words to search the Medline database. Which one, two or three words will you key in first? Then, which words will you add, and in what order, to narrow the focus of your search?

► Begin your search and key the words in, exploding, combining and modifying the search according to the order of key words you have just specified and the numbers of papers you obtain at each stage. Go back to the instructions about using Medline and work through the examples and helpful suggestions if you have difficulties doing your own search.

► How did the search go? Print off the results of the search in the same way as the tables given as examples earlier listed the stages of the search, the modifications and the numbers of papers identified from the key words. If you cannot print the results off the screen, copy it down over the page under the sub-headings 'Set', 'Search' and 'Results' as in the example tables.

Set	Search	Results
1		

▶ When you get down to less than 20 or so articles, scroll through the abstracts on the screen and print off the details of the ones that seem most relevant. Write down up to five sets of details of articles that seem relevant, giving article titles, authors' names, year of publication, volume of journal/source and page details.

▶ If you have still not obtained any relevant evidence you have a choice of trying other databases, or following up references given in papers with content nearest to your field of enquiry, or contacting experts named as authors or investigators to find out if there is work in press or other publications you have missed, or any other pertinent information.

You should not expect to find exactly the same details as in the examples given earlier as not only will you have modified the problem, the linked question and the search strategy to fit your own circumstances, but the details of publications held on the Cochrane and Medline databases will have changed over time.

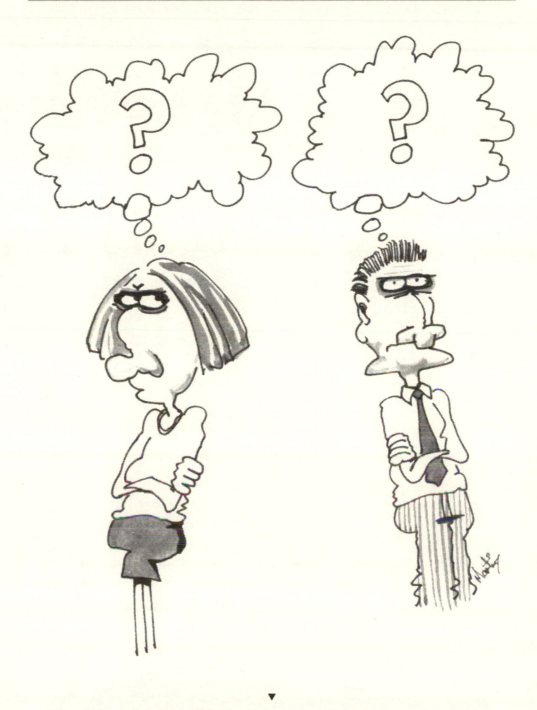

Choose a question that is important to you and your colleagues at work and where changes in practice will be possible.

Frame your own question and search for the evidence

Now that you have learnt the theory behind doing a search and have seen how other health professionals like you have framed their questions and searched for the evidence, you should be ready to shape your own question and find the best available evidence that exists.

1. Think about a problem at work which you consider would be an appropriate topic for this exercise. Consult others at work, do they think it is a problem too? Is it an important issue for them and do they think you would be spending your time wisely searching for evidence about best practice? Is there likely to be a change that you could make which would bring benefits to you, colleagues or patients, or result in a saving of resources? As this book is considering how to improve clinical effectiveness you should choose a clinical topic in this instance, but another time you might choose to search for evidence on a management issue. What is the problem you have chosen to investigate? Write it down here:

Who else did you consult before deciding on this problem?

What sort of changes at work do you have in mind that might be possible to put into action, depending on what evidence you find?

2 Frame the words of your question which address that problem. Build up the question as described previously, being as specific as possible, but not so specific that you narrow your field of enquiry and eliminate possible options that might be appropriate, such as novel types of interventions. Include the purpose of the question, what it is about, the setting, the population and the outcome(s). Write in your own words what the question is:

Are there any subsidiary questions?

Have you discussed the question with anyone else? If so, with whom?

3 Choose up to five key words and put them in order of priority:

Are you satisfied that these key words reflect all the essential ingredients of your original problem and capture the essence of the question?

4 Undertake a search for the evidence to answer the question. If possible go to your medical library and book time with a medical librarian and the computerized search facilities there. If the library has Cochrane and Medline searching facilities, try the Cochrane database first and then Medline.

Cochrane search

▶ Write down how you will use your key words to search the Cochrane database. Which one, two or three words will you key in first? Then, which words will you add, and in what order, to narrow the focus of your search?

▶ How did the search go? How many 'hits' did you obtain from the Cochrane database?
  – systematic reviews on the Cochrane Database of Systematic Reviews (CDSR):
      (i) number of reviews =
      (ii) number of protocols =
  – controlled trials on the Cochrane Controlled Trials Register (CCTR) =
  – abstracts on the Database of Abstracts of Reviews of Effectiveness (DARE) =

▶ Write down up to five sets of details of articles that seem relevant to your question, giving article titles, authors' names, year of publication, volume of journal/source and page details. Print off the abstracts of these articles if you are able to do so. Obtain copies of the original papers.

Medline search

▶ Write down how you will use your key words to search the Medline database. Which one, two or three words will you key in first? Then, which words will you add, and in what order, to narrow the focus of your search?

▶ Begin your search and key the words in, exploding, combining and modifying the search according to the order of key words you have just specified and the numbers of papers you obtain at each stage.

▶ How did the search go? Print off the results of the search in the same way as the tables given as examples earlier listed the stages of the search, the modifications and the numbers of papers identified from the key words. If you cannot print the results off the screen, copy it down here under the subheadings 'Set', 'Search' and 'Results' as in the example tables.

Set	Search	Results
1		

▶ When you get down to less than 20 or so articles, scroll through the abstracts on the screen and print off the details of the ones that seem most relevant. Write down up to five sets of details of articles that seem relevant, giving article titles, authors' names, year of publication, volume of journal/ source and page details.

▶ If you have still not obtained any relevant evidence you have a choice of trying other databases, or following up references given in papers with content nearest to your field of enquiry, or contacting experts named as authors or investigators to find out if there is work in press or other publications you have missed, or any other pertinent information.

Save your search on a floppy disc before logging off so that you can come back to where you were if you want to continue to modify the search upon later reflection.

STAGE 4

Appraise the evidence

Now that you have extracted the publications that seem most relevant to your own question from your search, the next steps are to decide how much reliance you can put on their contents and how far you can extrapolate from those papers to your own circumstances. This will involve deciding whether the studies described in the papers were well conducted or flawed, whether the population and setting studied were similar enough to your own circumstances for the results to be generalizable to your population or setting, whether sufficient people or things were studied for the results to be representative of larger numbers, and how you will weigh one paper against another if they report conflicting results or conclusions.

Critical appraisal is the assessment of evidence by systematically reviewing its relevance, validity and results to specific situations.

Critical appraisal:

- identifies the strengths and weaknesses of a research paper
- develops a better understanding of scientific principles and research methodology
- increases capability to understand to what extent published literature is applicable to other circumstances.

The meaning of different research methods and terms

Confidence intervals

This describes the degree of confidence that can be placed on any statistical result. It describes the range of results from the subjects or things studied within which the investigator is 95% certain that the true population mean lies (the usual level of confidence chosen).

Controlled trial

As for a randomized controlled trial (see relevant entry) without the randomization element.

A controlled trial detects associations between an intervention and an outcome but does not rule out the possibility that the association was caused by an unrecognized third factor linking both the intervention and the outcome.

Incidence

The numbers or proportion of new cases of a disease or condition occurring within a population over a given period of time.

Intention to treat analysis

This is a quantitative estimate of the benefit of a therapy in the population being studied derived from comparing control and treatment groups.

Numbers needed to treat (NNT) are being cited in published papers increasingly commonly. You need to know the characteristics of the population being studied, the disease and its severity, the treatment and its duration, the comparator and the outcomes.

Meta-analysis

This is a method of combining two or more studies to obtain information about larger numbers of subjects. Inclusion criteria should be clearly stated in the method to enable different studies to be considered together. It should appear reasonable to treat the sum of the different studies as one whole and that like is being combined with like.

Observational study

There are several types of study where the subjects are observed over time and the experiences are recorded or reported.

A cohort study is one where two similar groups of people who do not have the disease or condition under study are observed prospectively over a predetermined period to see the effects of one group being exposed to an already established suspected risk factor (such as cigarette smoking) and the other group not being so exposed.

A cross-sectional survey gathers information about subjects or things in a study population at one point in time or over a relatively short period.

Power

Sample sizes should be calculated before the study design is finalized to determine the numbers needed to be likely to detect a sufficient effect from the study intervention, so as to be sure that the effect did not occur by chance alone. The power calculation predicts the number needing to be studied to detect an effect at least at the level of 95% significance. This is the level of certainty that is equal to or less than a one in 20 risk that the effect occurred by chance and was not due to an intervention or event being studied.

Prevalence

The proportion of 'cases' within a specified population at a given time.

Probability

Probabilities are often written as p values in published reports where p stands for probability. It is a measure of how likely an outcome is. This lies between 0 (where an event will never happen) to 1.0 (where it will definitely occur).

The p value is a guide to the likelihood that the outcome measured occurred by chance or was due to the intervention or event that the study was designed to measure.

A significant p value is one where the likelihood is that the effect or outcome occurred as a result of the intervention or event being studied, and did not occur by chance. The most common convention is to decide arbitrarily on a one in 20 risk of being wrong about the direct causal relationship between the intervention or event and the outcome; that is, the risk that the outcome occurred by chance. This can be described as '$p = 0.05$', 'at the 5% significance level' or as a '5 in 100 probability' that the outcome occurred by chance. If written as '$p < 0.05$' there is less than 5 in 100 risk of the outcome having happened by chance. Smaller p values give increased confidence in the test results; for example $p < 0.001$ indicates that the probability that the outcome occurred by chance is less than one in a thousand. The level of significance the investigators choose should depend on the importance of being right about the intervention/outcome relationship, and the numbers in the populations being studied.

Sometimes investigators get carried away, testing every bit of data in their study to see if they can dredge up some significant results. This is very bad practice because even a short questionnaire can yield hundreds of combinations of possibilities if each question has several alternative categories of answers, for example age might be subdivided into nine decades. If a significance test was applied to all the possible combinations of answers looking for potential links and 200 tests of significance were tried, for example, you would expect ten tests erroneously to indicate statistical significance where the outcome(s) had occurred by chance (that is, 5 in 100 risk $\times 2 = 10$). So the arbitrary $p < 0.05$ test of assumed significance is not cut-and-dried proof that an outcome is directly attributable to an intervention – it is just a good indicator of significance.

Randomized controlled trial

Randomization is necessary to minimize and, hopefully, eliminate selection bias. This is the type of study design which is most likely to give you a true result because only one section of the subjects or things in the trial are exposed to the intervention or factor being studied. The subjects or things are randomly allocated either to the group exposed to the intervention or to the control group who are not intentionally exposed to that intervention. The experiences and outcomes of both groups are compared to see if they are significantly different according to statistical tests. Sometimes the design includes more than two comparative groups.

Using the randomized controlled trial method distributes unsuspected biological variables equally between the two groups, as well as any other external factors of which you are unaware. Both the subject and control groups will be exposed to these unrecognized external influences (called confounding factors) and any differences in outcomes between the two groups should be attributable to the intervention being studied.

When the term 'randomized' is stated there should be some information in the method as to how this randomization process was carried out to minimize any external influences from interfering with the random allocation of subjects or things to different arms of the study.

If a trial is 'double blind', neither the clinician/investigator giving the treatment or analysing the results, nor the person receiving it, should know whether they are in the treatment or the control group. In a 'single' blind study, either the clinician or the subject knows what treatment the subject is receiving.

Relative risk

Relative risk is calculated by taking the ratio between two measures of risk. If there is no difference between two groups the risk ratio is '1' as the risks in each group are the same. A risk ratio greater than '1' shows the outcome in the study group to be better than that for controls.

The risk ratio is the proportion of the group at risk in one group divided by the proportion at risk in a second group. The risk ratio is a measure of relative risk.

Reliability

A reliable method is one which produces repeatable results.

Sensitivity

The true positive rate of a diagnostic test, that is, how often the test misses people with the disease.

Specificity

The true negative rate of a diagnostic test, that is, how often the test indicates people as having the disease when they do not.

Systematic review

Systematic reviews of randomized controlled trials provide the highest level of evidence of the effectiveness of treatments – preventative, therapeutic and rehabilitatory treatments (as described in the section on hierarchy of evidence, pp 37–8).

Validity

A valid method is one which measures what it sets out to measure.

Reading a paper

Reading and evaluating a paper is mainly about applying common sense. Traditionally, critical appraisal of the literature has been made to seem like a difficult science for the elite, rather than a basic skill that any health professional can readily learn and apply to their own situation.

If you read the summary of a research study overleaf and answer the questions you will soon discover for yourself some of the common flaws in published studies, sometimes even those in respected peer-reviewed journals where the mistakes were not noted by the researchers or publication team.

In general you should consider whether:

▶ the paper is relevant to your own practice
▶ the research question is well defined
▶ any definitions are unambiguous
▶ the aim(s) and/or objective(s) of the study are clearly stated
▶ the design and methodology are appropriate for the aim(s) of the study
▶ the measuring instruments seem to be reliable; that is, different observers at different points in time would arrive at the same outcome

▶ the measuring instruments seem to be valid; that is, the investigator is actually measuring that which she/he intends to measure
▶ the sampling method is clear
▶ the results relate to the aim(s) and objective(s) of the study
▶ the results seem to be robust and justifiable
▶ the results can be generalized to your own circumstances
▶ there are any biases in the method of the study
▶ there are biases in the results, such as non-reporting of drop-outs from the study
▶ the conclusion is valid
▶ you have any other concerns about the study.

Specifically you should look at:
▶ where the study was done and who are the authors
▶ the study design: how were the subjects and controls selected, were they randomized and if so how, what were the outcome measures, were the outcome measures clinically relevant, are the sample numbers appropriate?
▶ the results: are the numbers of drop-outs and non-respondents reported, are all subjects accounted for, is the statistical analysis explained, are the results clearly presented?
▶ the discussion and conclusions: does the report describe the study's limitations, are the conclusions supported by the results?

Critical appraisal of a published paper or report of a study

1 The aim(s) and /or objective(s) of the study should be stated clearly.

  ▶ The aim should state the purpose of the study succinctly and specifically. It should be set in the context of information that is already known from previously published literature.

▶ The reasons for, and need to carry out, the study should be justified in the introduction of the paper.

▶ There should be a clear route built up from the aim to the conclusion flowing from the explanation of why a particular study design, population and setting were selected, to the results reported, the discussion and interpretation and final conclusion(s).

2 The methodology should be appropriate for the aim of the study.

▶ Quantitative and qualitative design techniques are complementary. A good quantitative survey will be based on prior qualitative work to determine what are appropriate questions to ask in the questionnaire or interview schedule. A randomized controlled trial may be a gold standard quantitative study design, but a qualitative method will most probably be needed to report people's observations, reflections and judgements.

▶ As a generalization, prospective recording is more likely to be accurate than retrospective recall.

▶ A sample of a population should be selected for study which is as representative as possible of the whole population.

▶ A setting should be chosen for a study which is as representative as possible of the setting of the total population to which the results of the study will be extrapolated.

▶ The sample size should be justified by a *power calculation* determined prior to starting the study based on the expected findings.

▶ There should be a method for increasing the response rate to as near as possible an ideal of 100% of the subjects included in the study.

▶ Details of any measurement or intervention should be as specific as possible, and transparently valid and reliable.

▶ A good study design will include a method to validate the questionnaire, rating scale or results obtained.

▶ It is always a bonus to see an original questionnaire even if only in an abbreviated form, to be able to judge for yourself the validity of the questions used in the study.

▶ The statistical methods should be described so that when the results are reported readers can check the statistical calculations and understand how the results were derived from the original data, if they wish.

3 The results should be robust, justified and related to the objectives of the study.

▶ The results should be simple to understand. It should be obvious where the results have come from and they should not seem to have been plucked out of thin air. Graphs and tables help to avoid strings of numbers and percentages.

▶ Statistically significant results should be presented in a conventional way or explained with full references if less well known statistical tests are used.

▶ Percentages should add up to 100% and if they do not there should be some explanation to account for the missing numbers. It should be clear where and whether subjects have not sent back the questionnaire, have left a particular question blank or given a 'don't know' response.

▶ If the results obtained from the subjects are fairly crude, such as when people are asked to estimate their answers or recall happenings in the distant past, the result should be given as whole numbers or to one decimal place, rather than given as several decimal places which might look more scientific to the casual reader.

▶ The written contents of a research paper should be in their correct places. Bits of method should not crop up afresh in the results, nor should discussion be interspersed in the results. The flow of the paper should be logical and build up to a justifiable conclusion. Anything otherwise is confusion and muddle.

▶ A low response rate may mean that the results from the sample of the population studied are not likely to be representative of the whole population. The further you regress from a 100% response rate the more likely it is that you have missed people or things that would give your results a different slant. As a very rough guide, a response rate of 70% seems generally to be regarded as reasonable for a topic where the results are not going to have dire consequences if they are wrong. But if the study was a trial of drug therapy where peoples' lives might be at stake if the research results and conclusions were wrong, anything less than a 100% response rate might be unacceptable.

4 Any biases in the design and execution of the study should be minimized and their likely influences acknowledged and explained.

► Good response rates are important because responders may have different characteristics from those of non-responders.

► There may be confounding factors present. These are so-far undetected influences that were not measured or recorded in the course of the study, that were actually wholly or partly responsible for causing the changes or results reported. There are often cultural changes with time outside the study and beyond the control of those undertaking the investigation. For instance, if a famous celebrity claimed benefits for a new treatment that was being studied, many more people would suddenly believe they had received the same benefits and the outcomes being studied at that time would be distorted. Opting for *randomized controlled trials* avoids the influence of con-founding factors.

► The potential and actual biases of the study should be openly described and their likely effects discussed in the Discussion section of the paper. Readers should then be able to make up their own minds about the relative importance of each bias on the results and how much the biases prejudice the extrapolation of the results to the readers' own situations.

5 Is the conclusion valid?

▶ The conclusion is often found in the Discussion section of a paper when there is no separate Conclusion section.

▶ The conclusions of the results should not hinge on probability test results. The significance of the results claimed should make sense from clinical and common sense perspectives too. For example, an intervention might claim that it is significantly better than another at increasing small children's height by 0.1 inches. But if, clinically, this difference is inconsequential, then the benefits of the treatment claiming to be superior are not proven by the positive significant result.

▶ The conclusion(s) should not make any claims that have not been justified previously in the report of the study.

▶ No new information should suddenly crop up in the conclusions that was not previously cited in the method, results or other section.

▶ It should be clear what the main findings mean and the implications for current practice or future developments.

▶ The results of the current study should be compared and contrasted with others reported elsewhere and any discrepancies interpreted and discussed.

6 Any other concerns about the study.

▶ Conflicts of interest should be stated, such as the sponsorship of the study by a manufacturer of the medication tested in the study.

▶ Look for any omissions in any section of the report. Think whether the implications from any contrary results seem to have been considered in full or glossed over.

Examples

Critically appraise this example – a summary report of a research study.

1 An investigation of the use of sunscreens in the United Kingdom

Summary

Aim: To investigate the use of sunscreens in children.

Method: A postal questionnaire was sent out to all 942 members of Women's Institutes throughout the Scottish Isles, asking them about the frequency of the use of high-factor sunscreens applied to their children (please contact the author for a copy of the questionnaire). Questionnaires were anonymous to ensure confidentiality. An article was placed in the Women's Institute newsletter to prompt non-responders.

Results: 356 women replied (85% response rate; average age 56 + SD 16.4298 years). 290 stated that they bought factor 10 or higher sunscreen. 89 preferred the scent-free version ($p < 0.1$). 350 women thought that the government should subsidize the cost of sunscreens as they were too expensive ($p < 0.0001$). The presence of a melanoma should be treated as a criminal offence and the sufferer fined for not having used sufficient sunscreen, as a contribution to the costs of the ensuing NHS treatment.

Conclusion: If the government were to subsidize the cost of buying high-factor sunscreens, uptake would be increased and the frequency of melanomas or other skin cancers would fall.

Source of funding: Nibblea Suncreams.

Conflict of interest: None.

Chambers R (1998) *J Evidence-Based Spoof.* **3**: 12.

Consider the following challenges

Write down your answers then read the author's opinion below:

1 Are the aim(s) and/or objective(s) of the study clearly stated?

2 Is the methodology appropriate for the aim(s) of the study?

3 Do the results relate to the aims(s) and/or objective(s) of the study? Are the results robust and justified?

4 Are there any biases in the design and execution of the study?

5 Is the conclusion valid?

6 Are there any other concerns about the study?

Critique of the summary report: use of sunscreens in the United Kingdom

1 Are the aim(s) and/or objective(s) of the study clearly stated?

The aim is not very specific. If the focus of the conclusion on cost of sunscreens and the impact of sunscreens on the frequency of cancers were intended as the purpose of the study then the aim has been expressed incorrectly.

2 Is the methodology appropriate for the aim(s) of the study?

No, no, no! There is already confusion as the aim and conclusions are so far apart, but working on the premise of the aim stated in the summary of the study given:

▶ the population chosen for study is inappropriate as children of Women's Institute members probably range in age from 1 to 60 years old; this can be deduced from the subject's average age being 56 years and the standard deviation (SD) of 16.4 years indicating that about two-thirds of the population studied are between 40 and 70 years (that is, 56 – 16.4 years = 40 years to 56 + 16.4 years = 70 years)

► the Scottish Isles setting is in a part of the United Kingdom that would be expected to have relatively low amounts and strength of ultraviolet rays, and results from this setting cannot necessarily be generalized elsewhere

► members of Women's Institutes living in the Scottish Isles whilst the study was in progress had not necessarily lived there all their lives; so if the geographical area was important the mothers do not have uniform histories of where they lived when younger, and their children may have lived apart from their mothers at any time previously

► the differing age range of the children means that some mothers' reports will relate to children under the age of 18 years currently receiving modern types of high-factor sunscreens, and others will relate to middle-aged children who may or may not have had old-fashioned creams applied a varying number of years previously; high-factor sunscreens did not exist at the time the study began

► there is no logic in choosing Women's Institute members as the population group to be studied – it may introduce a further bias if it were shown that members were more likely to be part of a more affluent section of society than the general population as a whole and therefore more likely to take holidays abroad where the sunshine was more powerful and potentially damaging

► mothers' recall of the frequency of use of suncreams applied to children up to 50 years before is unlikely to be accurate

► anonymous questionnaires that do not bear a code number make chasing up of individual non-respondents impossible – an article placed in a newsletter is unlikely to be an effective method of encouraging non-responders to reply.

3 Do the results relate to the aim(s) and/or objective(s) of the study? Are the results robust and justified?

It is obvious that the results are inaccurate and meaningless. Also:

▸ the response rate was very low at 38% (356/942), not 85% as stated
▸ the results, such as the information about costs of sunscreens, are not related to the data that would have arisen from the study method described
▸ it is ridiculous to give the standard deviation (SD) to four decimal places when the average age is given as a whole number
▸ a probability of < 0.1 is not significant and no such conclusions can be drawn about a proportion of the population studied preferring the scent-free version
▸ results should be factual and not offer interpretations, as here where the government is encouraged to treat the presence of melanomas as a criminal offence
▸ the results cannot be generalized.

4 Are there any biases in the design and execution of the study?

The study is riddled with biases from start to finish. Many have been described already, such as:

▸ the nature of the population
▸ that retrospective recall of information is likely to be poor
▸ the poor response rate
▸ the changing nature of commercially available sunscreens over time throughout the study
▸ the fact that the conclusion does not relate to the rest of the study, which implies that the whole purpose of the study may have been to prove that sunscreens should be subsidized and that the design and reporting of the study might be biased to that end.

5 Is the conclusion valid?

No it is not. It does not follow from the rest of the report and is not related to the original aim.

6 Are there are any other concerns about the study?

Although the author of this report states that there was no conflict of interest, the sponsorship of the study by a manufacturer of suncreams should alert readers to scrutinize the report even more carefully than usual for possible biases.

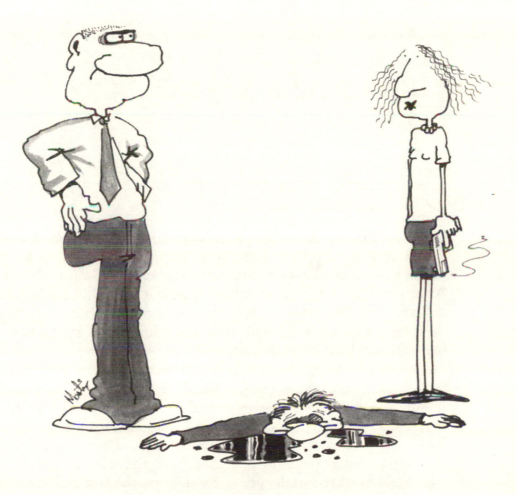

▼

Remember that sometimes the evidence can be misleading.

Critically appraise this second example – an unpublished report of a research study. Answer the following challenges, as before – write down your answers then read the author's opinion:

1 Are the aim(s) and/or objective(s) of the study clearly stated?

2 Is the methodology appropriate for the aim(s) of the study?

3 Do the results relate to the aims(s) and/or objective(s) of the study? Are the results robust and justified?

4 Are there any biases in the design and execution of the study?

5 Is the conclusion valid?

6 Are there any other concerns about the study?

2 An investigation of prisoners' health compared with that of the general population

Introduction: Recent work has shown that prisoners are disadvantaged in terms of their social background, their health status and the quality of health care they receive (Smith 1984; Walmsley *et al.* 1992). Research carried out in Bedford prison (Martin *et al.* 1984) found that prisoners had tended to neglect their health before reception into prison and 46% had active medical problems at admission.

Many of the people sent to prison have mental health problems. Gunn and others (1991) found that 37% of sentenced prisoners sampled from prisons in England and Wales had a psychiatric disorder, 2% of whom were suffering from a psychosis that was being inadequately treated and required transfer to hospital. A further 15% were thought to require additional treatment at the prison for their psychiatric problems.

The suicide rate amongst prisoners is several times that of their peers in the community and is rising disproportionately to the increase in the prison population (Dooley 1990). In 1992–93 (Wool 1994), 27 male prisoners committed suicide and in addition there were open verdicts on ten other males who died. The number of recorded incidents of self-injury is also rising steadily – 2612 prisoners were reported to have injured themselves on 3281 occasions in 1992–93 (Wool 1994).

A recent review of prisoners' physical health (Adam 1994) reported an increased incidence of alcohol problems, epilepsy, peptic ulceration, hypertension, hepatitis B infection, tuberculosis and self-neglect (skin infections, caries). Alcoholism is ten times more common amongst new prisoners than in the general community and 86% of new prisoners smoke (Martin *et al*. 1984).

This study set out to compare lifestyle habits of inmates in six prisons in the West Midlands with general population norms and measured prisoners' general health using the SF36 health measure (Jenkinson *et al*. 1993).

Method: Between 50 and 61 prisoners in each of the six prisons were surveyed between March and August 1994. Prisoners were interviewed in private rooms by the research associate. All prisoners thought to offer a potential security risk and those residing in punishment blocks were excluded from the study. Fifty prisoners were recruited in all establishments except one prison where 61 prisoners were chosen to allow sufficient sampling of the remand as well as the convicted men, and a second prison where 60 men were selected when two blocks of prisoners were demarcated for the study.

The method of selection varied according to individual prison procedures. In three prisons, clerical staff did not allow access to lists of prisoners' names and prisoners were recruited by a volunteer system. In the fourth prison all 60 inmates on education and physical education courses were interviewed. In the fifth and sixth prisons, every tenth inmate was selected from the list of inmates. Prisoners who refused or could not be interviewed were replaced by volunteers.

The interviews were conducted in a private room in which only the researcher and inmate were present, or a quiet corner of a large room. The inmate was assured that any information given was confidential to the research team and that a report would not identify any individual prisoners. All questions were asked by the interviewer so that literacy was not required.

The interviewer asked questions about lifestyle, and administered the SF36 survey form (Saudi Arabian version) (Ware and Sherbourne 1992).

The question schedule was piloted on ten prisoners before the main study began. Questions were amended accordingly. The prisoners participating in the pilot survey were excluded from the prison population selected for the survey.

A Minitab statistical package was used for processing the data and analysing the results.

Results: Thirty-six of the total 381 prisoners invited to be interviewed did not attend because they were unwilling, had appointments elsewhere, were thought by prison staff to be unsuitable for interview for security reasons, were confined to the punishment blocks or refused to be studied.

The mean ages of prisoners interviewed are shown in Table 1. All were convicted prisoners except 24 of the 61 surveyed in one prison, who were on remand.

Table 1: Age of prisoners interviewed in the six prisons studied

Prison code number	Mean age of subjects (standard deviation)*
P1 ($n = 61$)	18.2 (1.5)
P2 ($n = 60$)	16.1 (0.9)
P3 ($n = 50$)	32.4 (11.1)
P4 ($n = 50$)	27.4 (6.5)
P5 ($n = 50$)	32.1 (9.9)
P6 ($n = 50$)	19.7 (0.9)

*Age ranges have not been given so as to preserve prison anonymity.

Table 2: Current smoking habits of inmates in the six prisons

Prison code number	Percentage of prisoners who were current smokers
P1 (*n* = 61)	90
P2 (*n* = 60)	82
P3 (*n* = 50)	82
P4 (*n* = 50)	88
P5 (*n* = 50)	60
P6 (*n* = 50)	90

Table 2 describes prisoners' smoking habits in gaol. Smoking was as common amongst young offenders as older adults. Less than five per cent of prisoners who had previously not been smoking had started smoking during their time in prison. There was a slight tendency for smokers to report that they smoked more heavily since coming to prison.

The majority of inmates (91%) in all six prisons exercised on three days per week or more. Six per cent of prisoners never exercised in five of the six prisons. Forty-six per cent of prisoners interviewed reported that they exercised more during their time in prison compared to when they were 'outside', 15% thought the frequency was about the same, and 38% thought they exercised less in prison.

All 321 prisoners who completed the questionnaire about lifestyle also answered the SF36 health survey. Table 3 gives the mean score for the eight variables of the SF36 and norms for a comparable group from the general population matched for age and sex, taken from Jenkinson *et al.* (1993). Prisoner means that were statistically different from general population norms are indicated in Table 3.

Mean SF36 scores for prisoners of all six prisons were significantly worse than general population norms for social functioning ($p < 0.001$ in all cases), mental health ($p < 0.001$ in five out of six prisons, and $p < 0.05$ in P4) and pain dimensions; in five out of six prisons, inmates had mean SF36

Table 3: Mean scores for eight variables of SF36 for prisoners from the six prisons and norms for a comparable group matched for age and sex, taken from Jenkinson *et al.* (1993)

Prison code number	Physical function	Social function	Physical limits	Emotional limits	Mental health	Energy/ vitality	Pain	General health
P1								
Age/sex match	92.8	90.2	91.8	82.9	74.8	66.4	86.6	72.0
Prisoners	97.5*	78.9**	80.0**	77.0	65.3*	57.3**	75.4**	67.3
P2								
Age/sex match	92.8	90.2	91.8	82.9	74.8	66.4	86.6	72.0
Prisoners	97.1	81.6**	73.8**	81.7	63.5**	49.3**	75.3**	68.4
P3								
Age/sex match	91.9	90.4	90.4	85.4	75.5	64.7	85.9	73.9
Prisoners	91.8	70.7**	78.5**	66.6**	65.2**	54.7**	67.7**	68.5
P4								
Age/sex match	93.1	90.7	91.6	85.1	75.3	65.2	86.8	74.3
Prisoners	93.7	72.9**	85.5	74.6*	69.4*	60.5	72.2**	66.1*
P5								
Age/sex match	90.2	86.6	86.0	80.2	71.5	58.8	80.8	74.7
Prisoners	81.2**	64.9**	76.0*	58.5**	53.5**	42.3**	54.5**	63.6**
P6								
Age/sex match	92.8	90.2	91.8	82.9	74.8	66.4	86.6	72.0
Prisoners	96.3	76.7**	84.0*	86.0	66.6**	59.4*	77.9*	66.9

Prisoner means that are statistically significant in comparison with the group matched for age and sex are shown by *($p < 0.05$) or **($p < 0.001$).

scores that were significantly worse than age and sex matched norms for physical limitations and vitality.

Discussion: This survey proves that prisoners have worse health and well-being according to a comparison with the general public using the SF36 scale.

The volunteers used in place of those prisoners who refused or were not allowed to participate in the study were suitable replacements as the interviewer picked subjects who worked in the same workplace or lived in the same prison wings instead. The chocolate gratuity received by prisoners who had satisfied the interviewer's questions was not considered to have biased the results.

Prisoners' exercise habits compared favourably with those of doctors, where 22% have been found never to exercise and only 16% to exercise at least twice per week (Chambers 1992). Far more of the prisoner subjects smoked compared to a third of adults in the general population (Health Education Authority 1989).

The SF36 scale is reliable, valid and acceptable. The numbers of statistically significant differences were startling compared to the general public's norms.

Conclusions: The general public is healthier than prisoners in the United Kingdom.

References for the paper:

Adam S (1994) *Learning across the walls: the prison service and the NHS*. King's Fund Centre, London.

Chambers R (1992) Health and lifestyle of general practitioners and teachers. *Occup Med.* **42**: 69–78.

Dooley E (1990) Prison suicide in England and Wales, 1972–87. *Br J Psych.* **156**: 40–5.

Gunn J, Maden A, Swinton M (1991) Treatment needs of prisoners with psychiatric disorders. *BMJ.* **303**: 338–41.

Health Education Authority (1989) *Strategic plan 1990–95*. Health Education Authority, London.

Jenkinson C, Coulter A, Wright L (1993) Short form 36 (SF36) health survey questionnaire: normative data for adults of working age. *BMJ*. **306**: 1437–40.

Martin E, Colebrook M, Gray A (1984) Health of prisoners admitted to and discharged from Bedford prison. *BMJ*. **289**: 965–7.

Smith R (1984) *Prison health care*. British Medical Association, London.

Walmsley R, Howard L, White S (1992) *National Prison Survey 1991*. HMSO, London.

Ware JE, Sherbourne CD (1992) The MOS 36-item short-form health survey (SF36) 1: conceptual framework and item selection. *Med Care*. **30**: 473–83.

Wool R (1994) Report of the Director of Health Care for Prisoners. April 1992–March 1993. HM Prison Service.

Critique of the report: an investigation of how healthy prisoners are compared with the general population

This critique picks out main points and is not intended to be comprehensive. The report concerns a real study that was carried out by the author but has been adulterated to illustrate learning points.

1 Are the aim(s) and/or objective(s) of the study clearly stated?

Yes, they are stated at the end of the introduction. But the bulk of the material set out in the introduction refers to the mental health of prisoners, whereas the aims imply that the study is mainly concerned with prisoners' physical health.

2 Is the methodology appropriate for the aim(s) of the study?

- ► The use of an interviewer for questioning prisoners seems appropriate as a considerable number of prisoners might be expected to be illiterate.
- ► There is no power calculation or indication of whether 50 to 61 inmates from each prison were valid sample sizes.
- ► The Saudi Arabian version of the SF36 might be inappropriate for measuring the health of a British population.
- ► It was good that a pilot study was undertaken to test the questionnaire and that those subjects were excluded from the main study.
- ► There is insufficient detail about recruitment and selection of prisons and subjects, administration and contents of the questionnaire for another researcher to be able to repeat the study in the future.

3 Do the results relate to the aims(s) and/or objective(s) of the study? Are the results robust and justified?

- ► There is an error in that the first line gives the total number of prisoners as 381 whereas the tables and other text describe 321 prisoners being invited to interview. This might indicate either a simple error in the report or an attempt to disguise the numbers of prisoners refusing to be interviewed.
- ► The table giving the SF36 results (Table 3) is very complicated and difficult to understand.
- ► There is no indication of what statistical test was used to calculate statistical significance and probabilities.
- ► Percentages rather than actual numbers of prisoners exercising were given so that it is impossible for the reader to check that the percentages have been calculated accurately.

4 Are there any biases in the design and execution of the study?

- ► There is no information about how the six prisons were selected nor how representative they were compared to others in the West Midlands or in the United Kingdom.

▶ The recruitment of prisoners by a mix of random selection and volunteers produced biased samples. The potential biases this created, if for example the volunteers were more health conscious, were not discussed anywhere in the paper.

▶ The prisoners' SF36 scores were compared with published norms for the general population. No account was taken of the likely different characteristics of prisoners with regard to previous level of education, literacy, occupational class, etc. and whether this might make comparison with average norms invalid.

▶ The method states that some prisoners were interviewed in a public room, throwing into doubt whether such interviewees would feel able to divulge sensitive information about themselves.

▶ There is no justification of why the SF36 was the scale chosen to measure general health of a prison population, nor whether it had ever been used for assessing prisoners before.

▶ Results for remand and convicted prisoners are mixed together with no indication of whether they are similar or why they are being combined.

▶ The 'chocolate gratuity' may have influenced prisoners in deciding to take part and in the answers they gave about their health.

▶ Comparison of prisoners' exercise habits with doctors and teachers does not make sense as they are such different populations.

5 Is the conclusion valid?

▶ No – the study has not proved that the general public are 'healthier' than prisoners. The results from prisoners in six prisons in one region in England cannot necessarily be extrapolated to the whole prison population of the United Kingdom. All the other types of potential biases to the results that are described above render such a conclusion invalid.

▶ The word 'healthier' has not been defined in the paper at all.

6 Are there any other concerns about the study?

▶ Information about chocolate rewards for completing the study is only admitted in the discussion and was omitted from the description of the method. Besides being wrongly placed, this raises suspicions about what else might have been omitted from the report.

▶ It is not clear why the researchers undertook such a study if they did not have officially approved access to prisoners' details.

So now critically appraise the report of a study you have identified from your search.

1 Are the aim(s) and/or objective(s) of the study clearly stated?

2 Is the design appropriate for fulfilling the aims – the population, the setting, the sampling technique, the type of study, the methods of measurement, avoidance of biases or confounding factors? Are all stages of the design described such that you could repeat the exact same study if you had a mind to do so?

3 Do the results relate to the aim(s) and/or objective(s) of the study? Are the results robust and justifiable? Can the results be generalized to your own circumstances? Are the results clear? Are there mistakes in the results?

4 Are there any biases in the design and execution of the study? Are they discussed in sufficient detail and are allowances made for their effects?

5 Are the conclusion(s) valid? What do they mean for your own practice?

6 Have you any other concerns about the study?

Critically appraise a review

Now that you have learnt to critically appraise a research report, try your hand at appraising a review. Refer back to the explanations about randomized controlled trials, probability, confidence limits or other scientific terms described in the earlier text if necessary. The same rules apply for carrying out a survey of all research about a topic as for individual research papers. The specific question being addressed must be stated explicitly, the subject population (relevant research reports) identified and accessed, appropriate information obtained in an unbiased fashion (by using specific criteria to identify which research reports should, and should not, be included in the review) and the final conclusions should relate to the evidence obtained from the research reports included in the review related back to the primary survey question.

Look particularly for information in the review to reassure you of the following:

▶ The topic and purpose of the review are specified.
▶ The search methods used to find evidence relating to the question should be stated. The review of the literature should be comprehensive – reasonable efforts should have been made to identify and include relevant studies by consulting a range of databases and tracking down 'grey' material such as that in books, from conference proceedings, consensus statements or annual reports.
▶ The studies included in the review should be relevant and appropriate to the main subject or issue being addressed.
▶ Only similar data have been combined from different studies with similar subject characteristics, circumstances and methodologies. The methods used to combine the findings of the studies included in the review should be stated.
▶ There should be enough details about the subjects, populations, settings and other important factors for you to be able to decide whether the review's results and conclusions will be relevant to your particular circumstances.

▶ The criteria used to define whether or not a study was included in the overview should be stated clearly in the methods section. The researchers should have adhered to those explicit inclusion criteria, avoiding any bias in their method of selection.

▶ The results should be presented clearly in a scientific way. The results should be understandable, numbers in tables should add up, and it should be obvious how any analyses were derived.

▶ The authors should describe how the quality of the papers was assessed – how many people assessed each paper, whether they were blinded to other researchers' opinions, what criteria of quality were used, whether these criteria were valid, reliable and reproducible, and whether they adhered to the criteria.

▶ The results should be relevant to the declared aim of the review.

▶ The results should be generalizable – the significance of different biases should be considered and their implications discussed. The author(s) should give a critical analysis of the scientific rigour of the studies in the review, with all interpretative remarks being justified.

▶ The results should be comprehensive. Negative as well as positive findings in the different studies should be described. The range of confidence limits gives more information than a mere probability statistic.

▶ The conclusions should be based on an overview of the data and/or analyses of all the studies included in the review.

▶ The outcomes should indicate clearly any modifications that should be made to future health care practice based on the evidence presented in the review.

An example of a published review has not been included here for reasons of space and because the same principles apply to undertaking a critical appraisal of a review as have already been discussed in the appraisal of the paper describing prisoners' health and lifestyles and the commentary would mainly duplicate notes on the prisoners' study.

If you want to practise your appraisal skills obtain a copy of the following review:

► Waddell G, Feder G, Lewis M (1997) Systematic reviews of bed rest and advice to stay active for acute low back pain. *Br J Gen Pract.* **47**: 647–52.

Read through the article first to get a feel for it. Then read it again conscientiously absorbing the details and making notes as ideas and concerns come to mind. Now use the checklist given above and work through the 13 checklist items, writing down your answers. The whole exercise should take you about three hours.

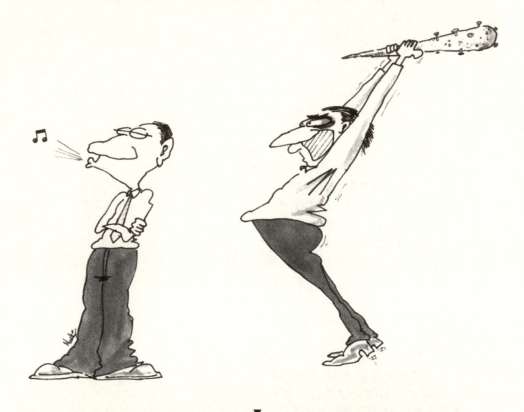

▼

It may be hard to convince your colleagues even when you've got the evidence.

Apply the evidence

You have identified your problem, posed your question with help from colleagues at work, searched for the best available evidence, judged the quality of the evidence, weighed the relative importance of any conflicting results, applied the evidence theoretically to your own circumstances and situation, and now you should be ready to apply the evidence in practice.

Clinicians have expressed concern about the dangers of adhering blindly to evidence in practice, and fears that evidence-based practice might be regarded as the be-all and end-all as far as decisions about the cost-effective delivery of health services go. Clinical judgement and common sense must be paramount in keeping evidence in perspective. The information forming the 'evidence' may be irrelevant, incomplete or inaccurate, or the 'evidence' may simply not be applicable in the particular clinical circumstances in question. The NHS has a long way to go in accumulating a bank of good and reliable information about current clinical care and best practices.

Sir Douglas Black[29] has recently warned about giving undue primacy to the evidence generated in randomized controlled trials. They may provide the best sort of evidence for evaluating the benefits of alternative medications, but they are not necessarily the best way of identifying evidence for resolving more complex human health issues.

Evidence-based management has an even weaker information base than evidence-based clinical practice. It must be right to encourage practice managers and other health service managers to adopt a research culture with a questioning approach. This will encourage them to reflect about what is happening, how and why, and to compare management practices.

So bear all this in mind as you think about applying the evidence you have gained from your search to your particular clinical situation. You may like to think of making changes from the perspective of an individual clinician, a practice or unit, or a Primary Care Group (PCG) or Trust.

Diary of your progress in searching for evidence

Complete this summary page of progress to date and your action plan for how you propose to introduce any changes in your working practices.

Write a summary of:

1 your problem (be as specific as possible so that you can measure the outcomes of any changes against this baseline position):

2 your question:

3 your search method – where you searched (databases, people):

4 the types of your best evidence (systematic review, randomized controlled trials, controlled trials, reports, conference proceedings, expert opinions):

5 give three titles of the most relevant and appropriate publications or sources that you found:

6 your conclusion(s) from the best evidence available in answer to your question:

7 the change(s) that you propose to make yourself or that others should make, as a result of the evidence you have obtained and the conclusion(s) you have drawn:

Action plan

People to whom you have fed back the results of the evidence:

Have you already written a timetabled action plan?   *Yes / No*

The baseline position:

Whom have you involved in discussions about the change(s) you propose?

Change(s) proposed:

People whom the proposed change(s) will affect:

Additional resources that will be required (people, premises, time, money, skills, etc.):

The timetable is:

Who will do what:

Advantages or health gains expected:

Disadvantages or losses that may happen:

How and when the changed situation will be monitored again:

Barriers to change

Once evidence has been gathered, projects have been completed and necessary changes discussed there can still be many barriers to overcome before worthwhile changes can happen.

The King's Fund PACE[6] initiative has identified the following barriers to change:

▶ others' lack of perception of the relevance of your proposed change (you should have realized this during your initial consultations with colleagues before you began)

▶ lack of resources to implement the change (time, staff, skills, equipment)

▶ short-term outlook of work colleagues

▶ conflicting priorities – without additional resources, changes have the potential to cause work overload or opportunity costs

▶ difficulties in measuring outcomes – it is difficult to find acceptable worthwhile health outcomes that are easily measured

▶ lack of necessary skills (forward planning is needed)

▶ no tradition of multidisciplinary working (this problem can probably only be surmounted with a culture change)

▶ limitations of research evidence on effectiveness (there's a lot more research about problems than there is about effective solutions)

▶ perverse incentives (a common flaw in the way the NHS functions)

▶ the intensity of others' contribution that is required (again consult early, get everyone on board and encourage everyone to 'own' your project).

And so …

▶ anticipate the strength of evidence you will need to convince your colleagues that the efforts and costs of change will be worthwhile – to them and the patients.

Read more about the lessons to be learnt in how to make successful changes happen.[6]

Starting to think about what clinical governance means

It is likely to be several years before the NHS realizes the full potential of clinical governance in promoting and maintaining quality. At the time of writing (mid-1998), people are only just starting to realize the meaning and implications of clinical governance, such as its potential importance in reducing inequality and making informed choices. Clinical governance is being seen as a balancing act between the control of professionals' practice and professional development, building upon quality control mechanisms at a local level. Hopefully professional self-regulation will continue so that clinical governance is professionally led.

Trusts are forming clinical governance support teams to lead on multidisciplinary practice development and take over the previous functions of quality assurance, clinical risk management, compliments, complaints and litigation, and clinical audit to meet their new 'legal duty of quality'.[30] This should focus chief executives and board members of Trusts as much on the quality of their clinical services as on financial matters. Clinicians should be better able to influence policy and planning of health care within the Trust and at regional and national levels of the NHS.

But clinical governance will apply just as much to primary and community care as to the acute sector. The extent to which the Primary Care Groups (PCGs) will be accountable for clinical governance will depend on their devolved level of responsibility for commissioning care, over and above the constituent practitioners' individual professional responsibilities. The various quality components of clinical governance cited by primary care leaders[31] include maintaining and improving clinical effectiveness, evidence-based medicine, clinical audit, complaints management, clinical leadership development, continuing medical education and continuing professional development.

The new performance framework, the local health improvement programmes, government and local priority areas and targets are all expected to be interweaved with the clinical governance culture.

As well as building on organizational influences of clinical quality, true clinical governance will not be achieved without the willing commitment of individual practitioners to high standards of practice. The key to high quality health care is good practitioner–patient interaction. All the other tools and measures listed above will not work by themselves and must be set up to support good front-line patient care.

In general practices, clinicians have always had the lead role in planning and delivering primary health care. And so the seeds of a clinical governance culture in primary care are already sewn. The main effect will probably be to increase the importance of evidence-based practice so that individual practitioners are more aware of recommended best practice and either adopt best practice or can justify why they are not doing so by citing clinical judgement or clinical/cost-effectiveness grounds. There will be more pressure applied to practices who fall below accepted peer-reviewed training practice standards. That pressure for best practice of clinical and management standards will be applied by internal standards of the PCGs who attain the higher levels of devolved responsibility for commissioning care. Poor clinical performance is usually due to contextual difficulties rather than because the erring clinician is intentionally 'bad'. Reducing the variability of standards in different practices and the primary care they provide may be helped by the unified budget and peer pressure within one PCG.

The Royal College of General Practitioners has broken down clinical governance into three distinct areas: 'the governance by clinicians of clinicians, the support of clinicians by managers, and the involvement of the clinician in the governance of the NHS'.[31] This underlines the need for a coordinated effort by clinicians, managers and politicians if clinical governance is to be meaningful. Clinical governance can only be effective if there are sufficient resources for clinicians to have the time, information technology and infrastructure support they need to identify, disseminate and apply the best practice that is affordable. Practice or PCG intranets, for example, may be the best vehicles for allowing all staff working for a practice, or all primary care providers within a PCG, to have access to the same, agreed, regularly updated treatment and management protocols, or accessing health-related web pages on the Internet.

Individual practitioners should start thinking about clinical governance in relation to themselves at three levels:

▶ their own personal and professional development
▶ their practice's or unit's development
▶ their PCG's or Trust's development.

Enhancing your personal and professional development

Continuing professional development should include gaining and refining knowledge and skills of high standards of practice. Good morale and significant job satisfaction are prerequisites of learning and effective working, and should be nurtured by targeted personal and professional development plans.

To be able to retain clinical autonomy and justify any of your management decisions that do not follow recommended guidelines or evidence-based practice will require you to have a more sure understanding of the facts than if you surrendered your rights to autonomy and blindly followed prescribed protocols.

Being well informed about best practice or the clinical facts will enable you, as a clinician, to continue to act as the patient's advocate, in patients' best interests.

Developing your practice or unit

This will involve the quality improvement processes arising from applying (clinical) audit, clinical effectiveness, risk management, multi-professional education, clinical protocols, monitored organizational policies, and appropriate changes, for instance in response to complaints or significant events. Patients' views and satisfaction with services should be a real part of your quality monitoring programme.

Leadership by a member of the practice or unit who accepts special responsibility for promoting clinical governance is probably essential in coordinating a strategy and gaining everyone's cooperation. That person will be responsible for keeping the others up to date on best practices, performance, new ideas for development, and overseeing training and resource needs with respect to clinically effective practice.

You should review the clinical guidelines that your practice or unit uses for disease management. Disease management has been defined as 'the development and implementation of treatment programmes for specific conditions in a systematic fashion to optimize the quality and cost-effectiveness of care using the best evidence available'.[32] Make sure that the guidelines are up to date and based on strong evidence. State clearly what section of your population the guidelines refer to. This may be a good time to invite patients to comment on the suitability of the guidelines. Ensure that staff are adequately trained for all tasks specified in the guidelines, especially for any skilled activities delegated by doctors to other staff.

Clinical governance in a Primary Care Group or Trust

Your information management and technology strategy will be the key to good communication and shared standards. For clinical governance to work across a PCG or Trust, it will require clinicians and administrators to collect data in uniform systematic ways to enable comparisons of efficiency and effectiveness of service delivery in different practices or units. Good IT services will be vital for linking clinical and organizational systems from across a PCG or Trust with the local health improvement programme to establish population and health needs, and monitor progress.

The clinical governance leader will need widespread support to keep the quality of clinical services at the top of the PCG's or Trust's agendas and in line with other organizations with whom they work in partnership at their interfaces.

There is bound to be tension between clinical governance and budgetary control, and it behoves clinicians to be well informed to be able to argue their cases for resources for staff, services and infrastructures.

Each PCG will need a team to lead on quality in general – including research, education, audit, and clinical governance. Hopefully the quality standards they set will be realistic and achievable, building on past developments, rather than result in a levelling down of the standards and efforts of better-performing practices.

Integrated care pathways are gaining popularity and will be one of the building blocks of maintaining clinical governance across the primary/secondary care interface. Integrated care pathways seem to work best if they are designed for a particular disease rather than a population. All health professionals who will be involved in executing the care pathway should be represented in designing it. Everyone's roles and responsibilities should be clear throughout the pathway. Monitoring how well patients' treatments adhere to the agreed pathway should reveal apparent gaps in care. These results can be fed back for the individual clinicians concerned to justify why their practice deviated from the pathway as part of the clinical governance programme and modify their future practice as appropriate.

Clinical governance will incorporate the recommendations from the National Institute for Clinical Excellence (NICE) and direct grassroots level implementation.

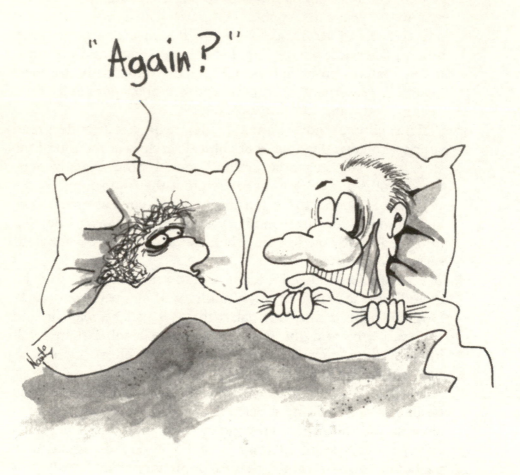

Once you've tried to apply clinical effectiveness – you'll want to do it again!

► EVALUATE YOUR NEWLY GAINED KNOWLEDGE AND SKILLS IN CLINICAL EFFECTIVENESS

Evaluate how much you have learned by doing this programme and compare your answers to questions 1 and 2 below with the equivalent questions in your initial self-assessment of your knowledge and skills about the topic at the beginning of this book.

Please circle as many answers as apply or fill in the information requested.

1 How confident do you feel *now* that you know enough about clinical effectiveness to be able to:

ask a relevant question?	*Very*	*Somewhat*	*Not at all*
undertake a search of the literature?	*Very*	*Somewhat*	*Not at all*
find readily available evidence?	*Very*	*Somewhat*	*Not at all*
weigh up available evidence?	*Very*	*Somewhat*	*Not at all*
decide if changes in practice are warranted?	*Very*	*Somewhat*	*Not at all*
make changes in practice as appropriate?	*Very*	*Somewhat*	*Not at all*

2 Which databases(s) have you used in this programme?

Medline   Cochrane   Internet   Other (what?)

3 What level of evidence did you find in answer to your question (or main question if you posed more than one question)?

strong evidence from at least one systematic review of multiple, well-designed randomized controlled trials (RCTs)

strong evidence from at least one properly designed RCT of appropriate size

evidence from well-designed trials without randomization

evidence from well-designed non-experimental studies from more than one centre or research group

opinions of well-respected authorities, based on clinical evidence, descriptive studies or reports of expert committees

no evidence at all.

4 To whom have you given a report about the evidence you found?

Colleagues at work   Friends/family   Bosses (managers) or GP at work   Other (who?)

5 What is/are the outcome(s) of you asking your main question and finding the evidence?

Made change(s) to an aspect of work – if so, please describe what change(s) you have made or plan to make, who was involved in deciding to make the change(s), who is involved in the new change(s), whether you need any more resources or training, and how you will review the change(s):

Decided against making any change(s) to any aspect of work – if so, why did you decide not to make any change(s) and who was involved in that decision?

Other outcome – what?

6 How will you use your new-found knowledge about clinical effectiveness in the future?

7 What did you like best about the programme in the book?

8 What did you like least about the programme in the book?

► USEFUL PUBLICATIONS

Bandolier is published by the NHS Executive, Anglia and Oxford as a monthly newsletter that describes the literature on the effectiveness of health care interventions in a pithy style.[33]

Clinical Effectiveness Resource Pack is produced by the NHS Executive, and is updated regularly. It includes lists of contact details for many organizations, publications and other sources of information on clinical effectiveness. There is also information about associated publications – the *Effective Healthcare Bulletin, Effectiveness Matters, Epidemiologically Based Needs Assessments, Systematic Reviews of Research Evidence, Clinical Guidelines, Health Technology Assessments* and other relevant publications.

Effective Healthcare Bulletin These bulletins are produced by the NHS Centre for Reviews and Dissemination at the University of York. They are 'based on systematic review and synthesis of research on the clinical effectiveness, cost-effectiveness and acceptability of health service interventions. This is carried out by a research team using established methodological guidelines, with advice from expert consultants for each topic. Great care is taken to ensure that the work and the conclusions reached, fairly and accurately summarize the research findings'.[34]

He@lth Information on the Internet This is a bimonthly newsletter for all health care professionals published by The Royal Society of Medicine in association with the Wellcome Trust.[35]

Health Updates from the Health Education Authority. Topics in the series include *Coronary Heart Disease, Smoking, Alcohol, Physical Activity, Workplace Health, Child Health, Immunisation.* These are well-researched reference books on topical health issues.[36]

Books

Baker M, Maskrey N, Kirk S (1997) *Clinical Effectiveness and Primary Care.* Radcliffe Medical Press, Oxford.

Crombie I (1996) *The Pocket Guide to Critical Appraisal.* BMJ Publishing Group, London.

Greenhalgh T (1997) *How to Read a Paper: the Basics of Evidence-Based Medicine.* BMJ Publishing Group, London.

Jones R, Kinmonth AL (eds) (1995) *Critical Reading for Primary Care.* Oxford University Press, Oxford.

The King's Fund (1998) *Turning Evidence into Everyday Practice.* The King's Fund, London.

Kobelt G (1996) *Health Economics. An Introduction to Economic Evaluation.* Office of Health Economics, London.

Muir Gray JA (1997) *Evidence-Based Healthcare.* Churchill Livingstone, Edinburgh.

Ridsdale L (1995) *Evidence-Based General Practice.* Saunders, London.

Sackett D, Richardson S, Rosenberg W, Haynes RB (1997) *Evidence-Based Medicine.* Churchill Livingstone, Edinburgh.

Computer language

Internet acronyms:

AFAIK: as far as I know
AKA: also known as
BTW: by the way
FAQ: frequently asked question
FYI: for your information
IM(H)O: in my (humble) opinion
NRN: no response necessary
TIA: thanks in advance
TTFN: ta ta for now
WRT: with respect to.

► REFERENCES

1 NHS Executive (1996) *Promoting Clinical Effectiveness.* NHS Executive, London.

2 Hicks N (1997) Evidence-based health care. *Bandolier.* **4**(5): 8.

3 Sackett DL, Rosenberg WM, Gray J, Haynes RB, Richardson WS (1996) Evidence-based medicine: what it is and what it isn't. *BMJ.* **312**: 71–2.

4 Haynes B, Sackett D, Gray JM, Cook D, Guyatt G (1996) Transferring evidence from research into practice: 1. The role of clinical care research evidence in clinical decisions. *Evidence-Based Medicine.* **November/December**: 196–7.

5 Haynes B, Sackett D, Gray JM, Cook D, Guyatt G (1997) Transferring evidence from research into practice: 4. Overcoming barriers to application. *Evidence-Based Medicine.* **May/June**: 68–9.

6 The King's Fund (1997) *Turning Evidence into Everyday Practice.* The King's Fund, London.

7 McColl A, Smith H, White P, Field J (1998) General practitioners' perceptions of the route to evidence-based medicine: a questionnaire survey. *BMJ.* **316**: 361–5.

8 Samuel O (1997) Evidence-based general practice: what is needed right now. *Audit Trends.* **5**: 111–15.

9 Prescott K, Lloyd M, Douglas HR, *et al.* (1997) Promoting clinically effective practice: general practitioners' awareness of sources of evidence. *Fam Pract.* **14**: 320–3.

10 Paterson C (1997) Problem setting and problem solving: the role of evidence-based medicine. *J Roy Soc Med.* **90**: 304–6.

11 le Vann T (1998) Are we doing any good? *Monitor.* **4 February**: 19.

12 Kernick D (1997) Why GPs should be wary of evidence-based medicine. *Pulse.* **13 December**: 48–50.

13 Houghton G, Mendes da Costa B (1997) EBM: a multidisciplinary educational needs assessment in the West Midlands (unpublished). This is an internal paper intended for local circulation only. It is available from the Evidence-supported Medicine Union, 27 Highfield Road, Edgbaston, Birmingham B15 3DP.

14 NHS Executive West Midlands (1995) *GRIP Kit. 1995.* The GRIP Group, NHS Executive West Midlands.

15 Aggressive Research Intelligence Facility (ARIF) (1997) *General Information Leaflet.* The University of Birmingham, 27 Highfield Road, Edgbaston, Birmingham B15 3DP. http://www.hsrc.org.uk/links/arifhome.htm.

16 Royal College of General Practitioners (1993) Portfolio-based learning in general practice. A report of a working group on higher professional education. Occasional Paper 63. RCGP, London.

17 Treasure W (1996) Portfolio-based learning pilot scheme for general practitioner principals in South East Scotland. *Education for General Practice.* 7: 249–54.

18 Burrows P, Millard L (1996) Personal learning in general practice. *Education for General Practice.* 7: 300–5.

19 Millman A, Lee N, Kealy K (1995) The Internet. ABC of Medical Computing series. *BMJ.* **311**: 440–3.

20 The Cochrane Library. Update Software Ltd, Summertown Pavilion, Middle Way, Summertown, Oxford OX2 7LG. http://www.cochrane.co.uk.

21 Kiley R (1997) Medical databases on the Internet – part 2. *J Roy Soc Med.* **90**: 679–80.

22 Kiley R. How to get medical information from the Internet. *J Roy Soc Med.* **90**: 488–9.

23 Kiley R (1998) Evidence-based medicine on the Internet. *J Roy Soc Med.* **91**: 74–5.

24 Oxford Clinical Mentor is available from Janet Caldwell, Oxford University Press, Great Clarendon Street, Oxford OX2 6DP.

25 Muir Gray JA (1997) *Evidence-Based Healthcare*. Churchill Livingstone, Edinburgh.

26 Kobelt G (1996) *Health Economics. An Introduction to Economic Evaluation*. Office of Health Economics, London.

27 Rowlands J, Morrow T, Lee N, Millman A (1995) Online searching. ABC of Medical Computing series. *BMJ.* **311**: 500–4.

28 Greenhalgh T (1997) The Medline database. How to Read a Paper series. *BMJ.* **315**: 180–3.

29 Black D (1998) The limitations of evidence. *Journal of Royal College of Physicians of London.* **32**: 23–6.

30 Department of Health (1997) *The New NHS: Modern, Dependable*. The Stationery Office, London.

31 Royal College of General Practitioners' Council (1998) Meeting Paper: Clinical governance, March 1998.

32 Smith P (ed) (1997) *Guide to the Guidelines. Disease Management Made Simple* (3rd edn). Radcliffe Medical Press, Oxford.

33 Moore A, McQuay H (eds). *Bandolier.* Pain Relief Unit, The Churchill Hospital, Oxford OX3 7LJ. http://www.jr2.ox.ac.uk/Bandolier.

34 NHS Centre for Reviews and Dissemination, University of York, York YO1 5DD. Subscriptions and copies from Subscriptions Department, Pearson International, PO Box 77, Fourth Avenue, Harlow CM19 5BQ.

35 *He@lth Information on the Internet* published by The Royal Society of Medicine, 1 Wimpole Street, London W1M 8AE. Tel. 0171 290 2927.

36 Health Education Authority (1997) *Health Update* [e.g. *Sexual Health*]. Health Education Authority, Trevelyan House, 30 Great Peter Street, London SW1P 2HW.

► INDEX